中中中

Introduction

Triangle has entered the Chat

Ramadi: We've been waiting. We don't have leisure time like you.

Triangle: Not my fault, blame Hope. She sent me on a mission.

Ramadi: I know, I shot at you and "missed".

Triangle: That was your guys?

Hope: We can start if you're done.
Triangle: Who's first?
Cortez: Me.
Doc: It's another goddamn animal story.
Sumac: I like them, you're just mad because he's a better physician.
Doc: Studying animals and applying it to humans is sick.
Cortez: More of our guys live than yours, my medical skills are better.
Kant: You're still both murderers.
Dmitri: *Justified* murderers.
Kant: I think Divo differs.
Divo: Don't drag me into this.
Chris: Can we start?
Ramadi: Go ahead Cortez. Still a dumb name.

***

***

The Fog

At the highest points of the Andes live the flamingos. They reside at such great heights to escape the noise of birds lesser. It's said the spirit of the ancients lie within every adult flamingo. Regardless of the average population's perception of docility, there are indeed flamingos that cause disturbance for the others. Today, my story is that of a young flamingo by the name of Hermes.

Early in the morning a pink bird stamped at the ice that entrapped his foot.

"How the hell does ice even get here?"

A small group of elder flamingos looked towards the struggling young with a glare on par with the sun. Hermes shut his beak and tried to go back to sleep. He thought over the day's coming activities with boredom. First, the sun would rise, melting the ice of the shallow pond. The group would smash the remaining mush that encased their legs, and would march around searching for food. By noon, half of the group would be residing in the shade, while the younger would bask in the extreme heat that accompanies areas wed to the sky. When the sun was halfway down its afternoon arc, the flamingos would again return to the pond. The water would remain warm for little longer, after which the time where food moved came to an abrupt end.

Hermes, however, was not concerned with food. He was the son of the king's brother; so countless servants satiated all of his desires. The king made sure all of his family was well fed, and even did his best to ensure the same for other flamingos. While he was by far the best king the flamingos of the Andes had ever had, his likeability had waned with the years. Birds have fickle minds, and a perfect king made the group question their leader's motives. There had been talk of destruction lower down the mountains. Trees were falling and the frogs were dying. Was the king simply trying to take their mind off of the coming death? It was all too easy to connect the abundance and peace with a king who would betray all in the end. Within Hermes' father's mind, this was a certainty.

"You're uncle is nothing but a coward. He refuses to see or do anything about what's to come. If we all stay fat, death will surely find us." He would tell Hermes under the moonlight.

For the most part Hermes ignored his father. He had seen how good not only the king was, but how his entire family was goodness incarnate. The wife would spend hours collecting food with the servants, and the son would teach the young flamingos how to fly. Hermes frequented their company more than his own father's, for honey attracts more bees than vinegar.

This morning, Hermes was eager to see his extended family. His father had just left for an extended fishing trip around the Atacama. As the sun began to rise, the thumps of a thousand birds smashing their feet against the ice echoed around the small valley. Within minutes, a fleet of pink marched around the lake, in search for a morning meal. Older birds sat back and basked in the early morning heat, as later on it became deadly to them.

Hermes made his way across the pond to where aunt Ava was sitting.

"Where's your father?" she inquired.

"He just left for his yearly trip."

"That's a shame" replied Ava, looking somewhat sheepish.

Hermes had not yet figured out how to read people, let alone the female flamingos. To him, they seemed like a mysterious creature of which no one ever truly understood the answer. Yanked out of his thoughts by the sight of a giant bird approaching, Hermes said "How are you doing today, King?"

"Hermes, you know you don't have to call me that." The Flamingo King shook his head.

"George, you know Claus left this morning?" asked Ava.

"Indeed, he told me a few weeks ago. He always loved this trip even when we were kids. I plan on joining him on the last day. A king needs a break now and again."

"You're really going to travel into that hell hole?" cawed a soft voice. It was Rufus, the prince of the flock.

"It's the Atacama, not the jungle, son." Said George, attempting to assuage the fears of his cowardly child.

"Ah, so you acknowledge there is danger down there?" replied Ava.

"Not of the sort that can harm us." Hermes, while he liked his aunt, thought her to be somewhat like his own father. She enjoyed gossiping while fishing, and had recently been extremely fearful of the growing reports from the Amazon. The adventurous young, seeking to escape the grasps of their parents', would foray into the unknown green for large fish, to prove themselves as adults. As of late, many of them had not returned.

The group conversed for some time before hearing a shrill call come up the steep hills.

"Someone get help! Clause has been injured!"

Hermes began to fly toward the edge of the small basin. His love for his father was not strong, but he would never wish death upon him. A pair of pink appeared, struggling to carry another soaked in red. Hermes rushed down to give them assistance. He could see his father was barely breathing.

"We have to get him to Wingless!" cried Hermes. The flamingos, too tired to speak, barely made it over the lip of the valley before ten birds swarmed to pick up Claus. Collectively, they flew him over to the other side of the basin, and began descending toward the Amazon.

A faint warning followed them from George, "Be careful! It's dangerous."

Why didn't the King follow? Thought Hermes. The question was brushed aside when the group of ten picked up their speed.

Twenty minutes later, they reached a cave in the side of one of the mountains. The birds smelled the acrid black substance that constantly permeated Wingless' residence. Hermes shouted, "Sir, we need your help. My dad's hurt!"

Out of the cave lumbered a dark skinned, bipedal thing that claimed his kind was known as "man". However, the flamingos had taken to calling him Wingless, as that was the true dichotomy that separated the world.

The man said nothing and examined the injured Clause before him. He looked plainly at the birds, "If I heal this man, many more will suffer." This took Hermes aback. As any dutiful son would he replied, "I don't care, just help him!" Wingless went back into his cave and retrieved what Hermes' assumed to be medicine. The smoke coming from the cave grew a deep purple, and Wingless began to chant foreign sounds.

The flamingos sat for several hours and watched as Clause was revived on the cold cave stones. Wingless informed them the injury was the result of another of his ilk. Breaking temporarily from the chanting for rest, Wingless told them of the encroachment of man. He relayed to them the horrible nature, and how few had sought to restrain it.

"Why don't we fight back?" Inquired Hermes.

"For two reasons. First, you have tried to fight back, and failed. Take a look at your father. You will not win, no matter if the sky turns pink and descends upon the world. You cannot win. Secondly, while man's nature is evil, it is not for you to judge man as a whole. I too belong to the bastards down the mountains, yet I am here helping you. Our nature may be evil, but those of us considered greatest seek to master it."

Hermes was too tired to fully comprehend what Wingless was saying, but the words of the sage would live in the back of Hermes' mind for the rest of his short life.

The sun had long set on the Andes. The beautiful gold faded to a pink and purple skyline. The sky painted with the lipstick of the fading sun gave way to the pale white light that shone down upon the land. Across the jungle, animals began to stir. But high in the mountain caves the nightly mist began to settle into the cave. Hermes sat at the edge of the cave, alone. The rest of his companions had awkwardly taken their one-legged pose on the hard rock of Wingless' den. Hermes gazed upon the vast greenness, basked in the moonlight. On any other night, his view would be restricted to the grey brown peaks that surrounded his lake. Tonight he decided to take in a view of the vast world.

If only he had been reading the omens of the cosmos. The warning from the sage, the unrest down the mountains, and now, it seemed Hermes almost escaped his fate. Something deep within his mind stirred, triggered by the moonlight. To him, the moon's beauty had turned something awful. A sickly projection of an ailing world made Hermes' stomach turn. In his last moments, he would think back to this feeling, and wonder why he was blind to his impending doom.

Hermes awoke with the rest of the flamingos. On this day, the force of the sun had woken them early. Its heat gathering in the cave like a dragon ready to breathe fire suffocated the birds. Hermes opened his eyes and placed his other foot on the ground. Without water nearby, the birds felt as if the heat zapped them of all their energy. Long before they had risen, Wingless was standing over Claus, finishing the incantation. Hermes walked over to the man and stood above his own father. In a sense, his speedy actions had denied his father the flight to the afterlife, for better or worse.

Wingless turned toward Hermes and said, "You did the right thing, and you will suffer because of it. However, the moment you turn from your morality, your life will no longer be a tragedy; for you will have made it Hell."

Hermes, with nothing on his mind other than saving his father, said, "My life is inconsequential to that of his."

Wingless, with a much harsher tone replied, "If that's your view of life, then you have already fallen to the wayside. I shall pray you have a quick death."

With those final words, Claus began to stir.

The wisdom of Wingless was quickly forgotten as Hermes called for the other flamingos to come. Claus had yet to open his eyes, but ruffled his feathers and made pained sounds. Hermes asked his father, "Are you okay?" Only to receive no response. Over the course of the next several hours, Claus came to. He stood up, wobbling on his two skinny legs, and looked surprised.

"Why am I not dead?"

One of the older flamingos replied, "Wingless saved you."

"What? Why would you take me to one of them?"

"It was that or let you die, Claus!"

"Then you should have left me for death."

Hermes, overcome by emotion, embraced his father. Claus recognized the fear his son had harbored and temporarily dropped his guise of toughness.

"It's okay son, you can stop hugging me. I'm alive."

"I... I was scared you were gone."

"Well obviously I'm not. I love you, but please, it hurts when you do that."

Hermes let go of his father and stepped back. Claus told his son, "I want you to leave and go tell your aunt everything is okay."

"What about the King?"

"Oh yes, tell him too."

Hermes flew out of the cave and rose to the small valley at the top of the Andes.

Hermes was greeted by a horde of pink, wanting to know the events that had occurred. He regaled unto them how Wingless had brought back his father, mentioning the bizarre chants and weird smoke. However, he left out the man's prophecy, as well as the eerie moonlight.

From somewhere in the back of the crowd, Ava flew over everyone to stand next to Hermes. "Leave the boy alone" she commanded, "He just almost saw his father die." George, much to his wife's dissatisfaction, joined Ava's side and reiterated her points. The crowd grumbled, but obliged. Hermes' aunt took the prerogative and berated the young flamingo with the very questions she chastised the flock for asking. In the middle of the questioning, Hermes felt something rub against his leg. He looked down to see Rufus nuzzling his beak, trying to get Hermes' attention. "I'm happy he's okay" said Rufus. Hermes saw the innocence in the child's eyes, and they brought forth all the emotions Hermes had done so well to hold back. Tears streamed down his face, and he embraced his cousin. The whole time George put on a facade of love, one that Hermes had grown accustomed to. Hell, Hermes had often worn the same mask when conversing with his father.

The family sat and conversed for a while, waiting for the return of Claus. Not long after, pink wings lifted up over the rim of the valley. Claus and the other birds that accompanied him landed in front of the royal family. George went to talk to his brother but was interrupted as Ava ran into Claus's arms, lamenting her fear of his death the whole way. Claus pushed his brother's wife off and went to discuss something with the King. Hermes was given was a short nod of appreciation, or maybe simple acknowledgement, from his father.

Claus and George separated themselves from the group. As time had gone on, George had become more and more certain Claus would try something stupid. His brother's recent injury further cemented this notion. "Brother, you know I gave up the kingship, to protect the flock," said Claus. "I kept it under wraps, still you and I are the only ones who know."

"I know, Claus."

"Then why, won't you listen to your elder brother? Something is happening and we need to fight back."

I wonder if that fight is ours or one of your own making.

"Why? Why must we fight back? Because you were reckless in your fevered pursuit?" George grew angrier. While his demeanor around others was collected and calm, his sibling's words always managed to ruffle the King's feathers.

George had an issue with conflict. Growing up, his life had been inundated with such. The flock had virulent political strife in George's youth, and his life had come face to face with death on more than one occasion. Other than the threat of assassination, the young prince was constantly faced with the fact he could never be his brother. Despite the love his parents had for George, Claus would always be the one who became king. The internal conflict caused George to externalize his need for safety. He prohibited all but his close family and friends from leaving the valley. He wanted to remain enclosed in his cushioned garden, to try and escape from fate. Yet, even though Claus had given up his position as king, the damage to George's psyche had already been done. That's why, when Claus even mentioned going to war, George lost his mind.

"We are not warriors. We never have been. We never will be. What is this insane drive that makes you want to venture into danger? Our world here is perfect!"

"And has it always been such? The land has never changed, but if we were perfect then strife would never had arisen. You should know this. You can't cushion reality; some bastard will rip it to shreds just for the hell of it."

"No, they won't. That's idiotic and naïve. If the world is perfect, no conflict will arise."

"If that's your belief, this flock is led by a blind king."

"It's this blind king who can banish you."

"You won't. Though you believe the world to be safe, there are creatures out there who don't share the same love as us flamingos. You need me to protect you, as with any coward. And I must say brother, to decry strength while hiding behind that of others is the biggest hypocrisy."

"I will not here your slander. As soon as your wound is healed you need to go."

"And take your wife with me?"

Claus turned and walked back to his sister-in-law. George stood looking down over the lake. The sun bounced off its pristine surface, causing rainbowed reflections to scatter. Sounds of love and fear came from the group George and Claus had left behind. The same sentiments would be echoed only days later when Claus was carried through the valley to commemorate his well-lived life.

It took less than a minute for Claus to fly back. George questioned him, "What the hell do you want? I told you we will not fight."

"You will not fight, and you will doom us all, proclaiming peace during the inevitable slaughter."

"It is wrong."

"It is self-defense."

"It is still wr…" George's words became inaudible as Claus closed his leg around George's throat.

"Don't make me into a killer." Claus loosened his grip slightly, as if he was surprised by his own strength after the injury. "We have a few ways to proceed. First, you can renounce the throne and give it to me. I highly doubt this is what you want, so we can disregard that option. Second, we can have an election. Birthright in the flock has always caused strife. Seeing how both our children are unfit to rule, a vote for leader seems acceptable. Thirdly, and I really don't want this to happen George, is you refuse both options and I crush your neck right now. I'll give you a minute to answer."

While the brothers stared intensely at each other, they heard a strange sound coming from the edge of the cliff. Instantly, Claus let go of George and ran to the cliff. Climbing the steep walls, was Wingless.

Wingless put hand over hand. Foot over foot. He started his climb early in the morning, when the nighttime air still cooled the cliffs. He had only made this climb twice before. Once, during his initiation as a shaman, to meet the great flock of the heavens. The next, when he came to give his blessings to the new king. For most of his adult life, Wingless had lived between the terrestrial and the heavens. He remained a wise man for both the humans below and the birds above. However, as he grew into his old age, Wingless began to notice the growing brutality of humans. Conversely, the flamingos had become more docile. Understanding how to read the way of the world, Wingless contemplated the outcome of the growing dichotomy of power. Certainly, the flamingos had the advantage. Animals, when they try, can outwit, outhunt, and out-kill humans. Did that mean there was no difference between the flamingos and the humans? There are ten thousand ways in which we can divide ourselves, but is that really useful? Rather, we should look at the individual as a cog in the greater machine of the universe. Because some have accrued more power, does not mean we can attribute it to the fault of any one collective, bird or human.

By the time Wingless reached the top of the precipice he was greeted by the King and his brother. They immediately understood the significance of seeing the man make the journey that would kill almost all other bi-pedals. They greeted Wingless with a bow, which he waved off.

"There's no need for such formalities."

Claus was the first to respond, "Wingless, are you here to assist in some way? What malady has caused the healer to seek us out all the way up here?"

"Well, Claus, I believe the malady to be one of your kind's own making."

George got a word in this time, "What do you mean? We've done nothing to anyone and restrained ourselves to this valley!"

"That's the issue. You have become weak, you have not shown love."

"To be strong we must demonstrate kindness to the others of the world?"

"No, you should show others you can do so."

"This is not helping." Said Claus. "Yet, I concede you are still the King, George. The decision of what to do next is up to you." The sarcasm dripped from Claus' beak. His threats from earlier were as true as before.

"Our heads have reached to close to sky…it is time to lower them to the ground." Sighed George.

Hermes stood among the other flamingos waiting to see what would happen. It had only been days since he last saw Wingless, but the flock in its entirety had not seen him since George's coronation. All the birds stood in the glorified pond, where all important speeches were made. George, Claus, and Wingless walked down from the cliff and walked through the crowd of birds. A pathway of pink parted, the trio marching alongside one another until they reached the center of the water. Surrounded by the flock, Wingless began.

"I thank you again for letting me enter your territory. When I come, I feel a closeness with the sky. Today is not one to revel in the heaven's glory. I come to tell you this feeling of closeness has clouded your better judgment. As you sat in your garden, the world has become chaotic. Your inability to spread the order achieved here, has led to stagnation. Should this stagnation continue, it is only inevitable that someone, or something, will come along and smash it to bits."

Claus started next, "I shall make my opinion known before the King states his. His word carries more weight, and will sway your mind if I do not speak now. We have become weak. And in this weakness, we have let the world pass us by. The lake in which we stand is the birthplace of our many ages. George was coronated here. Our father was executed here. Our children birthed here. Yet, we have confined ourselves to these waters. There is a world outside to which we rarely venture. As time has passed, the world has gone to hell. Yet, we have confined ourselves to these waters. The increasing ferocity of the growing world will be insurmountable even when we unify as the flock. Yet, we have confined ourselves to these waters. I ask everyone, why is that? Why have we hobbled ourselves so? The tyrant of old forced us to stay in this valley, and now we willingly do it. What's the difference between being so terrified of the world we remain enclosed, and the tyrant being so terrified we may see the world, he encloses it around us? Why are we scared of doing things? Was it not the goal of the tyrant to keep us from the outside world? Why? Why would he do that? What potential exists in the outside world that can be manifested into something of which the tyrant is terrified? Each of you that contribute to the collective fear is the tyrant of our flock. But more importantly, you are the tyrant of your own mind. The world outside awaits us, yet, we have confined ourselves to these waters."

"What do you want?" Shouted someone in the crowd. The pin-drop silence was interrupted by the soft squawking of questions.

"I say that we fight. We have hidden ourselves for too long, the only option is to show our strength. I propose we push back the humans that have begun to encroach on these mountains. It is only a matter of time before they come. I will die fighting for the glory of the heavens and our flock. You may die standing fearful in these waters. Going to confront this beast is our calling. To refuse is to be a coward."

The flock erupted into a cacophony of opinions. Some cried their support for Claus, while others called him a terrorist. In the midst of the commotion sat Hermes, unsure of what his thoughts were. He temporarily put them away and continued to observe the situation.

"SILENCE" commanded Wingless. The birds fell silent as the shaman's bass shook the valley.

"I shall speak next." Said George. "Claus is in part right. We have become too docile in our word. Our actions have become those of an infant, however, that does mean we should turn into killers. My brother has accused me of softness, but where he sees red I see a chance to make peace with a useful adversary. We can use the humans as protectors, to ensure we will have our continued peace at this lake. In return, we will allow them to visit this valley when they want. This plan is so simple and obvious my brother's objections are nothing short of obtuse. Who actually wants to fight?"

Hermes listened to his uncle's comparatively short speech. It appeared as though the King already knew it was a lost cause.

"But, I know this is not the general will of the flock. You want to fight. I can no longer mediate our issues. For that reason, I am resigning as King, and appointing my nephew, Hermes."

"WHAT?" shouted Hermes, Claus, and everyone else in the valley—except for Wingless. But once the clamoring reached a suitable level he began to speak.

"Hermes, stand before me." Hermes walked through the crowd toward the center of the water.

"From these waters has come all of existence. From this valley you have formed your garden. As a king, it is your right to do what you want from this garden. And now, I bless you with the order that should be with you in times of crisis."

Wingless performed some hand motion and place his hand on Hermes head. Scooping up some water in his hand, Wingless then said. "And now, I bless you with this primordial chaos. So that in times of strife you may have the creativity to overcome all obstacles in your path. The edge of these two elements is where you must live, should you seek to be a good King."

The flamingos stood in a stunned silence. Hermes was beyond that. In his mind he briefly recalled the lethargic paleness of the night not so long ago. But, the collective roar of a thousand flamingos tore through the valley. It mattered not that Hermes was young. Not that he was the nephew of the King when the King had his own rightful son. Not that he had no experience beyond the single trip to the shaman's cave. The only thing that mattered was that George had declared him king.

Hermes looked around the swarm of pink to find his father. In what appeared to be a genuine smile, the father beamed brightly. Hermes had rarely seen his father demonstrate love, and knew better than to trust his first instinct. However, the energy permeating the air drove out any thoughts of trouble.

That night Hermes sat surrounded by the elders of the flock. George and Claus were also there.

"King, your father, myself, and one other are heading out soon to take count of the enemy. Although we do not agree on the way to proceed, knowing our foes' number is useful information."

"Why are you telling me this?"

"Because, Hermes, you are now the King."

"Please, uncle, stop calling me that."

"My boy, I am proud, albeit mildly jealous, of your position. I'm sure your uncle just wants to show you the respect you showed him." Said Claus.

"Is there anything you wish for us to take special note of on our mission?" asked George.

"Uh, not that I can think of. Be safe, please."

"We will, son."

Hermes stood in the lake reflecting over all that had occurred in the past several days. His father had almost been killed, was brought back from the underworld, Wingless climbed the mountains, and Hermes was now King. Other than the impending decision he would have to make regarding the human issue. In the end, he would most likely default to George. Under his rein, no one got hurt. It would be naïve to change that. Hermes closed his eyes and began fading away into sleep.

All of a sudden, cries of "help" and the thump, thump, thumping of the other birds mashing the ice woke Hermes from his slumber. What the hell is going on? He thought. Quickly, he began smashing the ice that surrounded his one leg to see what had occurred. A group of flamingos walked toward him and the lead one stated, "Sir, you must remain here. Something terrible has happened and we can't have you lost in the confusion."
"I'm going to see what happened."
"Then we shall be your escort."

The same paleness of the earth lay upon the mountains of the Andes. The sun would not come for several more hours, and the disease would thicken, continuing it's choke of the Amazon. On a ledge a little below the rim of the valley, stood a flamingo. Beside him, a crimson red mixed marred the pink feathers of a dead bird. Hermes flew down next to the lone flamingo and said, "Where are my father and my uncle?"
The bird looked at the ground.
"WHERE ARE THEY?" Hermes' emotions were riding high when his lead guard nudged the King.
"Sir, they were attacked by a raiding party of humans. These two were the only ones to make it back, and this one the only to live."
"Are you saying they are dead?"
"No sir, but there is an undeniable chance that it is the case."
"Then we're going after them."
"Sir, I can't let you do that. I have strict orders to keep you here."
"I'm the one who gives orders now." Hermes turned to the still stunned flamingo, "Take me to where the attack happened."

The soft flapping of wings seemed quiet compared to the noise of the jungle. During the night, all that laid still rose like creatures from some undead army. The flamingos were awake, but the Amazon was aware, ready to hunt.

The birds that embarked on the scouting journey were 5 in total. Claus, and two of his compatriots, along with George and one of his fellows had left late at night. Of the flamingos that returned, George's friend was the one who lay bloodied on the cliff's edge. For the past several hours, George's friend, named Rosen, led the group to a clearing. As pink feathers descended from the canopy, they were surprised by the dark crimson that splattered a clearing.

"We were among the branches, looking down on a group of them. They appeared to be resting, with one standing guard at the edge of the firelight. We prepared to take off when something knocked Gil out of the tree. Immediately, Claus attacked the assailant. The wingless that launched the arrow was directly below us. He had managed to hide himself within the floor of the jungle. As the bow thummed the man hooted for the others to wake up. Claus was grabbed, and although he continued to peck, he was subdued, and I lost track. I have no idea what happened next. I fled as soon as I saw Claus head down. We had discussed beforehand that should anything happen, the King, er, the old King and Claus would cover the other three's escape."

Hermes observed the scene with disgust. His emotions remained during the journey but let go of their grip on the mind. When Hermes arrived, he managed to rationally (if not exactly calmly) examine the situation. Around the clearing, there were no bodies. However, as the group spread out a little, Hermes discovered a trail leading away. He was by no means the best tracker in the group, and so called everyone over.

"I think we can follow this."

Rosen responded, "Gil didn't die here. That means someone lived."

"No shit" replied the lead guard. "But, that doesn't mean it was one of us."

"Doesn't matter. I say we go."

"Sir, plea-"

"No." Hermes was beginning to see the usefulness in the power of kingship.

The group followed the trail, guided by the lead guard. Blood dropped a path on the lush jungle but was barely visible and the thick foliage above blocked the moonlight that permeated the clearing. The flamingos could only tell the way thanks to the darkness that covered bright plants.

"When what's inside comes out, it stains the world." Said Rosen.

"Where'd you get that one?" inquired Hermes.

"Just an observation."

"Is it really a stain if what is black lays itself bare?"

"Yes, evil is evil is evil."

"Let's consider different realities before blanketing the world with 'observations'."

"Sir, with all due respect, you two are far too loud. We should remain quiet and track." Chastised the lead guard.

"You're right, my apologies Areon." Replied Hermes.

The group continued following the bloodstains by what Hermes discerned could only be some deep seeded instinct. A few hundred more paces down the red road, a slight bit of pink emerged from the undergrowth. Hermes knew better than to run, it might be a trap. But keeping in check the need to disregard surroundings was a difficult task.

In the darkness to the left, something began to stir. A form darker than the night that enveloped the jungle ran past the group and grabbed whatever had been lying on the ground. Hermes could no longer hold back, he flew full speed in pursuit of the demon—the rest of the group behind him.

Hermes flew full speed until he reached total isolation. His speed had carried him far away. He knew the group would eventually catch up, but for now he remained isolated. Looking around, Hermes noticed little. The fog that lay upon the jungle had descended into the trees. A silvery gray mist infected the rainforest. In the gray shade, Hermes saw a darkness slink. It was slow. A methodical hunter took slow pace after pace around the lone bird.

Although he was tracking the shape with his eyes, Hermes' vision barely registered the panther. It leapt with deadly accuracy at the flamingo. Through sheer luck, Hermes managed to flap above the tiger's grasp. But, he knew he wasn't much safer. In the trees lurked worse things. Even then, the cat could easily nab the new king. The spirit of his father inhabited him; concerns for safety were dropped. If I am to die regardless, I'll do so in-

The panther had ripped Hermes' throat, and the now dead king had passed. From somewhere in the mist, another shape emerged.

"Thank you, James. It needed to be done." Said George. "I couldn't do it any longer. Claus would certainly have killed me, taken my child, and my wife for his own."

"Whatever you say, sir."

"Where are the rest of the lot?"

"Taken care of."

"That's not an answer."

"You have no more need to fear for your life from your fellows."

"Then I have no need to fear."

"Whatever you say, sir."

Interlude 1

Hope: That was dark.

Diog: Not compared to what you guys do.

Dmitri: We're the good guys.

Kant: I'll keep saying how you were a bad student. You can't reasonably call people good or   moral.

Ali: I thought it was a good story Cortez.

Divo: I liked it too. But you did just kind of rip off Shakespeare.

Cortez: Everyone rips off Shakespeare.

Triangle: Who's next?

Diog: We're using this random generator thing right?

Doc: This is why we left. You don't know basic technology.

Diog: Yes, I'm sure societal recession occurred because some old people didn't fully understand   technology.

Sumac: Singapore's doing just fine over here.

Doc: Cuz you don't have old people running the country.

Hope: Diog! What's the story today?

Diog: A great tale about how rebellion is full of narcissism.

Avenging Socrates

Heath lolled over in his bed, exhausted from yesterday's proceedings. He had attended the façade of a court in order to support his friend. They both already knew the outcome, but the bastard hadn't bothered to defend himself. Instead, Socrates attacked his accusers. Heath still wasn't sure why. The audience was on his side, until he critiqued them for being sheep.

Socrates was sentenced to public execution in a week. Heath had visited his friend early in the morning to plead for him to escape. To stay seemed antithetical, Socrates was one of the greatest minds to ever grace the earth. His wisdom and public debates attracted people of all ages from all areas. But now, he'd rather die than prolong his existence.

From Heath's understanding, the only reasons Socrates was staying was for sake of pride and because he felt an obligation to fulfill his duty for the city. Heath contested the principles on which he stood were pointless if it led to death. But what really made his blood boil was Socrates's belief he owed the city something. What had the city ever done for him?

Heath had trouble with this line of reasoning the most. As he stared blankly at his ceiling, his thoughts raced with counter arguments. Last I checked, you didn't sign shit. Not only that, you are a freeman. Your obligations are to those to whom you say they are. Your simple presence indicates nothing; fool. Do we blame the man who is murdered because he stood in the wrong spot? Goddamnit Socrates you're wasting your life.

The next few hours Heath spent in his bed contemplating what to do. Socrates was to be executed early next morning by the bastards who accused him of "corrupting the youth." The idiots can't see the 'corruption' Socrates caused was simply to allow people to actually think. No more indoctrination into the old ways; no more acceptance of what is presented by those above you. No, Socrates made people think for themselves. One of Heath's favorite moments lie when he utterly ruined the idea of power as justice. That day, Heath realized what a great man Socrates was.

The sun blazed down upon the town square. A crowd of three hundred had gathered in the sweltering heat to watch a forum between a poor man who had recently become famous for his ability to argue and the university headmaster.

It had taken months to organize this event. Initially, the headmaster had refused. His reasoning was Socrates would use underhanded tactics befitting one so uneducated. However, pressure from students and other academics eventually broke the man down, and he accepted to debate Socrates as long as he knew the topic of debate beforehand. This would give the headmaster, Polemarchus, a chance to prepare. Socrates agreed to these terms. Some took his confidence as arrogance, but when Socrates began deconstructing the man's arguments Heath realized that the confidence was more than earned.

The topic for today's forums was whether those who contribute more to society should be held to the same laws as those below. Polemarchus took the side of power, and began with a short speech:

"The mere fact that this is occurring will only serve to prove my point. Those belonging to the lower levels of society are integral to making life work. The farmer grows food. The warrior protects the walls. The cobbler makes shoes. Without them, our society would surely fall. But, our society will surely fall should these men, the farmer, the warrior, and the cobbler fancy themselves in the roles of others. Should the farmer think to fight, enemy combatants will beat him. Should the warrior try and make shoes, our soles would be bladed and impossible to use. And if the cobbler thinks he can grow produce, we would be chewing upon leather. These occupations are closer in origin than the beggar and the academics. The beggar manipulates others for wealth; the academics provide knowledge to increase prosperity for all. Should the beggar have to adhere to the same rules as the academic? You would have the beggar's words questioned instead of giving the poor soul a few coins? That's sickening. Before this debate begins I would just like to say you are making the lives of your fellow destitute only more difficult by showing your kinds' manipulative nature."

Socrates answered without missing a beat, "We beggars are known for manipulation? Can I be at fault if you confuse manipulation for truth? I have no qualms with holding my words to the same standard as yours."

The arbiter in charge of the debate chimed in. "Quiet down. The proposition today is the question of laws both moral and state. Should all freemen be held to the same standards? Out of respect for the graciousness of the headmaster to entertain this discussion, Polemarchus, you may go first."

Polemarchus nodded toward the arbiter and stood up. "We live in an unprecedented time. Wealth floods our city as the waters of poverty inundate foreign lands. Unfortunately, this wealth has allowed some to think they can entertain notions destructive to the very fabric of our society. Rules this city has created apply to citizens differently, this is well known. And, it is well known that this is rather useful. We charge guards fines should they show up for work late. Yet, we do not do so for the farmer. Why? It is not the farmer's job to show up on time, whereas it is one of the guardsman's main responsibilities. We fine the farmer if he doesn't produce enough food but not the guard. Why? It is the farmer's responsibility to feed the city, not the guard's. Now, we must apply this notion to our words. The ramblings of the insane are treated with little respect. Why? They're insane. Anyone can point out what babbling is, and it takes no intellectual prowess to debunk deranged ideas. However, there comes a time when the insane gather a following. The words of the intelligent can easily be confused with the words of the insane. Wealth displays the difference.

Would an intelligent man choose to be poor? No. Intelligence is demonstrated through the wealth one has accrued. Wealth does not necessitate intelligence, but intelligence requires the pursuit of wealth. This must be kept in mind when debating. If your partner has little wealth, it is likely his mind will be as small as his wallet."

Socrates smiled. "You seem to have forgotten the question at the end there. In your words, we hold the farmer to different standards than the guardsman. But, this is a falsehood. Would you hold different guardsmen to different rules?"

Polemarchus replied, "If all I am to do is answer your questions, I fail to see how you can win."

Socrates answered, "Then, sir, entertain the masses and answer the question by demonstrating my stupidity."

"No, all guardsmen are held to the same rules."

"And farmers?"

"The same."

"Then it seems your conclusion is not that we hold different people to different rules. Instead, you claim different jobs have different rules. This observation is obvious, but I congratulate you on stating it."

Polemarchus' voice grew irritated. "Fine. If you want to twist my words then we can play that game. The wealthy contribute more to this society. Wouldn't you say the king does more than the peasant?"

"No, not necessarily. But, for your point I will pretend the answer is yes."

"How dare you say a peasant is greater than our king. Do you not hear this heretic? And some of you claim he is the voice of reason. Ridiculous. Regardless, would you behead the king like a peasant if he stole from a merchant?"

"Absolutely."

"And here is where your intellectual deficit shows. The king gives more to society than the peasant. Those who give more deserve more, and thus, deserve to be exempt from certain rules."

"Was the king born?"

"Yes."

"Was the peasant born?"

"Yes."

"Will the king die?"

"Yes."

'Will the peasant die?"

"Yes.'

"Then I fail to see how societal contributions exempt one from the law. If we are all born of a woman, then we are all equal. The laws then, should apply equally. We are all created the same, and we all end the same. Why should our lives be treated as anything but the same?"

Polemarchus fired back, "You falsely equate the human condition to equality. We all are born and we all die, certainly. What you do in the time you are given is what truly matters. Those who give more have earned their keep, and thus, become the progenitors of society. Without them, society would fall into pieces so barbaric it would resemble the wild. If you are to shackle those at the top to the rules of the bottom, we would perish quickly and covered in blood."

"Polemarchus, why do we have laws?"

"To keep the peace and protect."

"Who are the laws meant to protect?"

"The people."

"Are the upper echelons of society not part of the people?"

"Certainly, they are. But in order to protect the most people these laws can be amended for the wealthy."

"Are all the wealthy equally good?"

"I presume not."

"Is murder always wrong?"

"To take the life of another without a valid reason is indeed wrong."

"So you cannot measure the good that is done, but you can measure evil? If an evil committed by a peasant is as bad as an evil committed by the king, why should it matter what good they've done? If the king was good in the past, it does not exempt his actions in the present. If a child is good for a day, and then fits the next, the child still receives punishment. If the same child promises to do good in the future, he still receives punishment for his crimes in the present. We are unsure of how to measure good, but we can measure evil."

Polemarchus was drug into minutia he did not comprehend. "We can certainly measure good. If a king gives a peasant some bread, it is far greater than the peasant giving the king bread. Both actions are in effect the same, but the king is demonstrating benevolence while the peasant is simply paying his moral obligations."

"Polemarchus, I would like you to give me a list of all possible actions and weigh them as good and bad."

"That'd be tedious, pointless, and insane."

"Then tell me by what margin are you measuring goodness?"

"By what is right."

"And, what sir, is right?"

"Any action undertaken by those who wield power, usually in the form of wealth. It is only through their benevolence that we are allowed to live, and so, it is through them we learn what is right."

"What is right is what the powerful feel?"

"Yes."

"You seem to be contradicting yourself. Earlier you claimed regardless of circumstance, murder is wrong."

"I thought the nuance need not be explained, so let me lay it out plainly for your simple mind."

"Please do."

"Murder is wrong depending on the murderer."

"The act is not what is wrong, but the person of the act?"

"Yes."

"Does that mean everything peasants do can be considered unjust?"

"What kind of backwards logic is that? Of course a peasant can do something right. Only, their just actions are more limited in number."

"And this is because the amount of good they do pales in comparison to that of the wealthy or the king?"

"Yes."

"You come back to this point consistently, although I think you don't quite understand the implications of such. You make the obvious assertion actions are wrong based on circumstance. But then you make the contradiction that an action's justness is dependent on the person doing the action. Somehow, the person doing the action is relevant to the circumstance. Only one who believes themselves greater all could make such a wild and destructive point. Polemarchus, you seem to miss the weight of an action is not measured by its outcome. If a farmer who has done all he can to produce crops in the fall, and a drought strikes, do we blame the farmer? In the practical sense he failed, but there was no way he could change the outcome. Yet, by your logic, this man is at fault for failing to bring forth food. As another example, imagine a city where everything is perfect. The king makes only just rulings, however you define it, and is his greatness basks the kingdom in glory. One day, while out walking, a man throws a tomato at the king. The king proceeds to execute the man by the regent's own blade. The kingdom won't suffer a loss, as the man was a beggar. Yet, the action is still wrong. What is moral is not only what is good for society. If that were the case, we would not be free to choose what is bad for society. The king should put people in their proper place, and if they stray outside, punish them harshly. Why, Polemarchus, is the action wrong?"

Polemarchus gathered himself and responded, "What is good for society is ultimately up to the king. If the king should choose to determine what is best for all is assigning occupations, then that is what is moral. Even if a king were not in charge, as in some neighboring lands, whatever the state decides is what would be right."

"You are wavering in your initial claims, seeing them disproven and resorting to other points. Again, I shall demonstrate why you are wrong. First, I must ask you, are laws and moral separate?"

"Quit your snipping at me peasant. Laws and morals are indeed separate. Morals are what we must defer to in the lack of laws."

"Then what are laws?"

"Bindings intended to restrict immoral behavior."

"So, the assumption is that restricting immoral behavior is inherently moral?"

"Yes, because all laws are inherently moral."

"I understand your point, I required only a yes or no in this instance. Your idea rests on the notion restricting behavior is a moral thing to do."

"How can it be any other way? My voluntary restriction to not strangle you is a moral thing."

"But therein lies the difference. You are choosing not to close those piggish hands around my neck. If a law necessitated that you not make an attempt on my life, would not doing so be moral?"

"Yes."

"Forced inaction or action is moral?"

The debate raged on for another thirty minutes, with Socrates deftly (if arrogantly) deconstructing Polemarchus' arguments. Eventually, the arbiter stood up. "Now, you have all heard the words of these two…men. It is time to pick a winner." Polemarchus' fists began to tighten in anger. "Who here, believes Polemarchus is the intellectual victory?" Silence. Not a voice was heard in the crowd of hundreds. It was as if the entire audience had their mouths sewed shut. The arbiter looked to Socrates. "Now, who believes the Socrates has won?" The crowd erupted in applause. Stories were told that the king's palace, a good several miles away, shook with the thunderous cheering. The arbiter eventually quieted everyone. "I believe Socrates to be the winner on this day. Polemarchus, that was a valiant attempt."

Socrates stood up and offered a hand to Polemarchus. "I'm sorry for the insults, I get caught up sometimes." Polemarchus spit in Socrates's face. "Your day will come. For every twist of words I shall tie another knot in your intestines. Lowly scum."

Socrates bent down and got right in front of Polemarchus' face, "I still won the debate, maybe try reading instead of fantasizing about getting inside another man." With that, Socrates walked down from the raised platform and was surrounded by people prospective students.

Heath waited until the sun sat upon the horizon. For hours, people had tried getting wisdom from Socrates. Heath just waited patiently. His occupation had developed this virtue well over the years. Often when guarding higher ups, Heath had to stand still for an entire shift, looking at absolutely nothing. At least here he could sit down.

The questions took until the full moon was about a quarter way up in the sky. Socrates indicated to those surrounding him that he required rest. Heath turned to go, if Socrates wasn't going to be left alone he could try and engage with the man on another day. Heath started walking when he heard someone say, "Man, why have you come here today?"

Heath turned to see Socrates looking directly at him. His disciples looked surprised. Why was their master talking to a random mercenary who hadn't even bothered to ask any questions?

"I heard there was a strange man in this town. I came to listen."

"Ah, but you already heard my debate. Yet, you remain."

"I found the questions interesting as well."

"You asked none. Why?"

"I didn't want to."

Socrates chuckled, "My friend, I would very much like to pick your brain. May I join you wherever you are heading?"

Heath stopped. He was staying at a tavern while he waited for some work. He supposed there was no harm in allowing the older man to tag along, although he wasn't sure if he would buy him a drink. "Sure, but don't expect me to pay for a mug."

"I would presume no such thing." Socrates got up and joined Heath. He turned to his followers and said, "My conversation tonight will not be of note, I recommend heading home, lest I bore you with questions that intrigue only myself."

"But master!" one of them shouted "All your dialogues are important! We should be taking notes on them all."

"Perhaps you should study your notes instead of blindly following the word of a beggar." Socrates seemed insistent, and the followers dispersed. Socrates turned back to Heath and asked, "Where are we going?"

"I forget the taverns name. I've spent too many nights in residences much the same. I'll know it by sight."

"Why rely on your sight? Surely it's seen the same taverns time and time again?"

"I can't help if my sight remembers. I just know it does, so I use it."

"That's a wise tactic, mercenary. If I am going to be sharing a drink with you, I'd like to know your name."

"Heath. And I'm not paying for drinks."

"You'd be surprised the amount of coin the acolytes give me. Tonight, is on me, for permitting my pestering."

"You are a con man."

"Do you believe that?"

"No. You twist words like the sophists do, but it's not the same. Actually, I think you are the probably one of the best word twisters I've seen."

"Oh?"

"You twist and twist their words until they no longer understand what they are saying. But you don't twist your own."

"I know my words to be correct, getting them to come to my point of view is difficult. I see the flaws in my own thinking. But, I believe the flaws to be less so. I use their words against them to point out the infinite cracks in their logic. Sometimes it's better to show why your opponent is wrong, than to prove yourself right."

Heath liked that saying. "Maybe your company won't be so bad tonight."

The pair reached the tavern just as the moon was directly overhead. Sound muffled by the tavern's doors reached out into the otherwise quiet street. People in this city tend to stay inside at night, thought Heath.

"Stay close to me so you don't get robbed." Warned Heath. "This place isn't known for its safety."

"I love danger as much as the next man."

Heath doubted the small man had been in a fight in the past two decades, maybe his entire life. He wasn't overweight, being poor provided a large barrier of entry. Socrates also wasn't in the same kind of shape you'd expect from someone who begged for scraps.

"Socrates, where do you spend your money?"

"On food."

"There's no way you spend all that on food." Replied Heath as he pushed open the bar's doors. A wave of heat and warm lighting immerse the pair as they stepped through.

"I don't recall saying it was all for me." A generous old bastard, thought Heath as they sat at a table in a darkened corner.

A bar maid walked over with a pitcher and asked, "Anything else?"

"That's all, thanks." Said Heath.

Socrates quickly interjected, "Actually, there is something I want."

"Unless you tell me what it is, I won't be able to get it." The girl said snar

"That's quite a harsh tongue for someone who works for tips."

"I have other ways of making money" she replied with a sly smile.

"I don't want that either. I doubt many other do."

"Pity, I always loved crotchety old men."

Socrates laughed, "May I have some bread?"

"Sure, one bread coming right up."

"A loaf, please."

"Indeed, you are." She smiled again, turned, and walked into the kitchen,

"Why do you have to torture people?"

"Was that torture? I think we both left with a smile."

"It was torture for me, I hate wordplay."

"Then why watch me?"

"Like I said earlier, you don't play with words. You twist and break the words of others. That, is what I enjoy."

"I think that's a rather normal human emotion. We love to watch things break. When the world becomes stagnant, we throw a rock at a window just to see what happens."

"You throw the rock at a window. I just enjoy the reaction."

"Why don't you pick up a rock and join me?"

Heath smiled for the first time since their encounter, "I've thrown too many rocks and broken too many windows. Eventually, you hit the person behind the glass."

"It is only one, why not continue?"

"For reasons you made earlier today. The life of the individual should not have rocks carelessly thrown at it. In fact, it shouldn't have rocks thrown at it at all!" Hadn't the old man argued for the sanctity of an individual life earlier that day?

"Have you killed anyone with these rocks?"

"Probably a few."

"The fault is not that you threw rocks, but that you threw them at the wrong window."

"How the hell am I supposed to know what the wrong window is?"

"It changes, just like you. Sometimes we should hit windows with people behind them, other times we shouldn't."

Heath sat for some time and thought. Socrates drained his glass of whatever swill the bar was serving. He refilled Heath's glass and his own.

"I think I have the answer."

"Oh? I wasn't aware I asked a question."

"To the whole window discussion, asshole."

"Enlighten the asshole." Replied Socrates as he continued to down beers. He remained sober despite the large intake of booze. That was something Heath could respect.

"We are using rocks as a metaphor for words, no?"

"Words, ideas, and the like, yes."

"Those in and of themselves cannot hurt people. Ideas do not hurt unless acted upon. For example, I may want to punch you in the jaw right now, but the act of thinking that has no bearing on reality. Thus, ideas without action are harmless."

"I concur."

"Then, distinguish between acting upon ideas and expressing them."

"Are they not one and the same?"

"Absolutely not. Expressing an idea can in no way be dangerous. If I express the idea that I think you are an old bat with a few tricks up his sleeve, you may feel insulted, but you suffer no physical harm."

"They say that the accumulation of mental harm creates physical harm."

"For certain it does, but many things cause mental harm. And, it is almost entirely subjective how the person will take it. For those too sensitive to handle words, they shouldn't engage with other people. It is not the fault of people throwing the rocks, because, in reality, those rocks hurt not everyone. Some rocks are bigger, some are smaller. Some hit their target, some miss. Some are intentionally thrown to injure, and others are thrown merely to create discussion. The subjectivity of the words is up to the individual, and it is not right to constrain the words available to others simply because someone, somewhere might get hurt."

"Ah, but is that not why we have laws? To prevent people from getting hurt?"

"The laws rely on theft on property, thus invalid."

"Well, that's another discussion for another day. I tend to like the state most of the time. But, I think you've shown yourself to be a bit of a liar."

"You dare call me such when I have a sword?"

"Why would you use your sword when you are so adept at words? You say that you hate the twisting of words, yet, you do the same."

"There is a difference between twisting words and speaking over booze."

"I grow tired of these conversations at times." Socrates said, downing another glass.

Heath remembered that first night very fondly. After a little convincing and negotiating over a salary, Heath became Socrates's bodyguard. The threats against him had been growing, and he needed the protection (he certainly had the coin for it).

The two spent the next several years travelling various cities, eventually returning to Socrates's hometown. He had grown older, and traveling was becoming cumbersome and damaging his health. Socrates's city went by the name of Grushow, and was ruled by a somewhat elected emperor, senate, and other various facets the provided a façade of democracy.

If only we hadn't returned. Nearly any city would have taken us, but he had to try and make a point.

Socrates had condemned himself to death. Heath still winced at recalling the events.

"Welcome! Today we have a now we have our very own renown scholar, and Senator Thrasymachus!" Announced the arbiter as the enormous crowed roared with excitement.

Half the cunts can't even hear what's going to be said, thought Heath.

"You will be debating the nature of morality. Socrates has elected to allow the Senator to go first, despite winning the coin flip. Senator!"

"Thank you, Socrates, I know many men have refused to debate you on the basis of your intellectual status. Of course, while yours may be great, it cannot compare to the education of the utmost elite. Thus, I must apologize in advance for giving you your first public loss.

"That aside, morality is nothing more than what those in power say it is. Look around. Do you see that? We construct the world with our hands. Does it not make sense that the construction of the metaphysical rests in the palms of creators? Who are the creators of morality? Objectively, I would think you to agree Socrates, morality is the law by which our mind should think righteous to act or not. The utmost expression of this rests in our democracy. Every so many years, we vote for our leaders. And what is voting other than expressing who we think to be the most moral candidate? Surely practicality goes to the wayside when we consider the moral nature of our leaders. The leaders, those with power, then become those who craft and change the law in accordance with what they deem to be moral. Law is simply the manifestation of what our leaders, and by proxy us, think is the most moral."

The arbiter announced, "Socrates, it is your turn!" The crowd that day turned unusually silent. By now the citizens loved him or hated him. Socrates was inarguably the most notorious public academic of the time. That day, Socrates's full intellectual prowess would be put on display.

"What part of your argument needs dissecting first? Ad hominems are wondrous tools for the small of mind, but I've grown tired of dissuading my opponents from using them. I commend you for limiting yours. Should you want to look a fool by debating me, I believe it your right.

"Regarding the first statement, we craft some of the world with our hands. We erect buildings and homes, aqueducts and theaters. Human reason has gone so far as to be able to create ideas we can discuss with others of our kind. But our ability to construct the world around us is limited by biology and the divine. To biology we are slaves who can manage small changes. To the divine, we are nothing but a clinging form.

"To make such an absurd statement about the nature of reality is to say that we are the constructors of the world is not only inane, but immature and atheistic.

"On the second point, you are attributing morality to democracy. Is that a decision you came to on your own? If morality is constructed by leaders and I reside in exile of all lands, who is the constructor of my morality? Would you claim I am still beholden to the laws that saw me rejected? No, of course not. The only way to actually determine morality is to imagine the lone man on an island. What does he have and not have in being alone? He has his person, his thoughts and his words. Nothing but death can remove the self from the earth. Now introduce another man, do they now have a new sense of morality? One can claim they now have a moral obligation to care for each other, if caring for each other turns out to be a benefit to the individual. Now, put families of the men on the island. Is there a new sense of morality? No. You can claim what is good for the family is only good if it is such for the individual.

"Suppose the families mutually decide to divide the island in half. The second family quickly runs out of food on his side and says he has a right to food of the first family. The families on the prosperous side of the island have no legal obligation to assist the other family. But, they must have a moral obligation—for to help the other is certainly to help the individual. In return for treating others with care and respect, the others have a contractual moral obligation to return the favor. This propels a cycle of goodwill.

"But, Suppose the second man's family intrudes on the first's side. The first man's family, as seen by his mere existence in nature, has a right to protect what is owned. Thus, if the family owns the land, they must too have a say of what goes on in that land. If a man intrudes, then a right to protection arises. After all, if the first man invaded the second's land, the expected response would be to protect.

"All of this morality comes down to one simple argument do not steal without justification. An entire moral code need only be constructed around this to effectively run a society."

Thrasymachus looked intrigued, an emotion often replaced by malice in many of Socrates's other opponents. "I must ask you Socrates, would you say moral and legal obligations are entirely separate?"

"Absolutely."

"And why my friendly peasant is that the case? The laws seek to enforce the morality you speak of. Should a man intrude on another's home, the law punishes the intruder in a way the individual cannot."

"To that I agree, the individual often lacks the ability to punish those who infringe upon his rights, especially concerning death. To this, I say a lawless society has a duty to protect its constituents. As for laws themselves, they can by no means be argued as moral, thus the use of them is inherently immoral. Laws require enforcement, and enforcement requires enforcers. These enforcers are paid by the state, and thus the state requires income. The only way for an entity to produce income is to create it or steal it. The creation of such income is an impossibility of the state, because humans create subjective value. As stated earlier, the individual is the one to create. Thus, the state requires theft to enforce laws, let alone other institutions such as the building of roads. One could say that the theft is justified from effect, for the theft results in greater good for the most amount of individuals, I would imagine this is your stance?"

Thrasymachus contemplated for what felt like an hour but was a mere second. "Can you call it theft if it results in a greater prosperity?"

Socrates replied, "And this is a part of the question of morality we have come to discuss. Can morals be determined by their outcome? This is only an example, although a useful one for framing this entire discussion."

Thrasymachus returned, "You claimed earlier what is good for the individual is how the determination of morals can be deduced. I question that statement. What is good for the individual in one instance, is not always good for the individual across all other instances.

"Take, for example, a drunken man. The act of wasting coin on a week on intoxication may be beneficial in the moment for forgetting his worries of the greater world, but would negatively impact him in the weeks, months, and maybe even years to follow through an addiction to coping with drunkenness. What is good for the individual may be what is good for all, but not if it sacrifices present welfare for that of the future."

Socrates smiled. "So what?"

The crowd collectively gasped. Heath's back grew a little straighter as he leaned in and paid greater attention. Socrates had asked his question with aggression.

Thrasymachus looked flummoxed. "What do you mean so what? Why does that not matter? You make no sense."

The arbiter looked confused and interrupted, "Does this mean the debate is…a draw?"

Socrates smiled, "It appears so!" The crowd looked more confused than anything. They expected a complete deconstruction of Thrasymachus. Part of what made people so attracted to Socrates was his takedowns of those who believed themselves better than the unwashed masses. Socrates took note of the general atmosphere and turned to the crowd.

"Why is there no applause today? Out of all the words I have exchanged publicly, these few have perhaps stood as the most important. If men cannot come to an agreement, there would be pointlessness in words. We would be nothing but brutes, killing to prove righteousness, rather than debating to discover true morality."

Some in the crowd cheered. Some in the crowd booed. Others simply walked away. Thrasymachus put offered a hand to Socrates, "Let us go back to my place and waste time contemplating more the ways of the world."

"I would waste my time no other way." Socrates refused the hand and motioned for Heath to follow. The mercenary walked up to the stage and looked Thrasymachus in the eye, "I don't trust you."

Thrasymachus nodded, "Acceptable. You too are welcome to my abode, if only to watch over this old man."

The feast was set for all who belong to the elite. Today, they came together in celebration of some stupid conquest. The victories abroad had begun to drive the powerful even more power hungry. They found looting other cities produced a steady increase of income, all while keeping taxes low. Money paid for in blood is often easier to hide than the theft of the populace. Heath's anger had only grown since Socrates's death, and these warlords became the epitome of what Heath had despised.

They had taken away Socrates, but it was not the death of the man Heath was upset about. Socrates was a friend, and Heath would grieve when his present task was fulfilled. For now, distracting emotions were thrown to the wayside. Heath's anger was derived from the very nature of these sub-humans. They were masters of death. They got rich from death. They employed death to kill dissidents. They used death as a tool to control the population. They were death, only fatter and drunker. Rather than wielding a scythe, they wielded the power of the law. Committing evil was below them. It was much easier to delegate it to those lower. Thus, the killers could abdicate responsibility. It was utterly despicable.

Heath had barely escaped the night of Socrates's death. Thrasymachus had put on a façade of intrigue, and a damn good one at that. He lured Socrates into his house and offered for Heath to come in. Heath insisted he would keep watch outside. After several hours, Heath saw two armored men approach him from inside the house. "Our master would like to see you."

"I answer to Socrates."

"Answer to death instead." The plated pair drew their short swords and lunged at Heath. Heath ducked under their blows and slammed his quarterstaff into one of their helms. The man fell dead. The second called, "We need help here!" Heath could hear more guards coming from the house. Heath had the option to escape; the house was ungated.

He stayed for another ten men.

Each time one came, Heath would crush their bones with his staff. He didn't understand what was happening, he didn't have to. Heath's fighting instinct took over, and he became lost in the battle. At one point, he could see Thrasymachus hurrying across the foyer, running to the back of the house.

Heath was slowly overrun. An onslaught of guards forced even the battle-hardened three time war veteran back. Heath turn to run and was confronted with another group of five guards running at him. Heath realized his only path out was through the house. Just as the guards converged and swung their weapons, Heath bolted to the nearest window and smashed it with the quarterstaff. He jumped through the window, getting only a few manageable cuts on his legs and arms.

Heath looked around what appeared to be a dining room. The crimson walls mimicked the anger inside Heath's own heart. Near the head of the table, a body laid slumped face first in a bowl of noodles.

Heath drove up to the gates and was stopped by the guards. "Why are you here sir?" asked a man with the list.

"Delivering wine for the party."

"Name?"

"Yara."

"I see." The guard checked his paper and nodded to the other at the gate door. "Go through."

The gates lifted up and Heath drove his horses into the courtyard. The grand hall stood apart from the rest of the palace. Of course, it wasn't actually a palace. Palaces were for despotic regimes; this king was democratically elected. That was the tale.

Heath had discovered at a young age that this was not the case, and wondered why no one else took notice. The same people won over and over again. And when they grew old, their sons and daughters to their place. In what world is that democracy?

Heath pulled around to the small kitchen on the side. He hitched Yara's horses to the post. He had convinced the young man he would deliver his wine with a pretty sum. Money was no object for Heath. Socrates had paid him well, and his wealth had exponentially expanded. The donations for Socrates were often given to Heath, as Socrates could usually live off the goodwill of others.

Only a man that great could ever accomplish such a feat. Heath was almost jealous. But now was not the time for jealousy, and Heath knocked on the kitchen door. A potbellied, sweaty cook in a dirty apron opened the door and asked in a rather annoyed voice, "What the fuck do you want?"

"I bring wine." Heath said in a peasant accent.

"YOU'RE LATE!" The cook exclaimed. "WE'VE BEEN WAITING, THE PARTY'S ABOUT TO START!"

"Apologies." Heath suddenly hoped the cook would die too, one less shitty attitude in the world. Heath held it together and continued, "Would you like me to bring them in?"

"YES! WE NEED ALL THE HELP WE CAN GET!"

Heath began to wonder if the man was deaf. Perhaps in return for serving the vile his hearing had been taken away. It didn't matter, Heath just had to make sure everyone drank the wine. If there was one thing the "elected" enjoyed, it was their wine.

He began unloading the barrels one by one and carried them into the kitchen. The cook announced, "NONE OF YOU SCUM ARE ALLOWED THIS UNTIL AFTER THE PARTY, I CAN'T HAVE DRUNKEN SERVANTS!" Heath changed his mind about the cook. Maybe he just hated his job. Making food for the worst of this world would harm the heart of even the most stalwart man. Many of the staff were slaves, their families threatened with death otherwise. The land had been on a downward spiral since a decade previous Socrates's death. Wars for alleged safety piled on top of a growing cultural ailment of disgust between fellow citizens. Without someone to speak out against the immorality of the world, those at the top found it easier and easier to suppress those who even implied it existed.

Punishment was death by execution, or death by joining the front lines. In either case, misery was certain. Only if one escaped to nearby lands was freedom possible. Even then, it was only a taste of what should be freedom.

Heath unloaded the last barrel and carried it to the kitchen. He asked the cook, "Can I stay for a while, my horses need to rest?"

"FINE! STAY OUT OF OUR WAY!"

"Of course, sir." Heath found an unused crate and sat down. This would be the most unpleasant part of the whole affair. He touched his short sword for reassurance, but the mind still wavered. Could he do it? Did these men deserve to die? Perhaps he should flip a coin again. Heath pulled out a copper piece and tossed it in the air. Tails for death, heads for life. Heath caught the coin.

After several more minutes the cook bellowed at the staff, "BRING OUT THE FOOD!"

Heath tried to keep his grin hidden. He watched as exotic foods from all around the conquered lands were carried out to the elite. If only he made them eat their own children. It was more symbolic. Suffering would come anyway.

Heath had spent two years travelling the world, looking for the correct supplies. He planned how exactly to take out the elected. There was no point in killing Thrasymachus on his own. He was not the originator of any assassination, multiple elected likely acted in tandem. Socrates's death was orchestrated. There was no other plausible way. Killings had to be sanctioned by the group. The public was never privy to killings. The wealthy could supposedly bribe the elected to choose who would be a target. Heath had spent months collecting these rumors before his travels. He had to analyze how the people operated.

During those years, Heath had discovered only he could judge their morality, God had no place on this plane. Heath had drowned days in the library, studying the great ideas and religions of old. Answers had to be out there in some dusty tome. Heath had learned from Socrates one's experience is not enough to determine the functions of the world. An undertaking into the ideas of others was necessary. He concluded God could not exist, and to believe in such is Ludacris. However, Heath could not negate entirely the possibility of the divine. Thus, it was required he justify his actions should he reach the end of the road and be deemed a sinner.

If God did exist, surely, he would be fine with these deaths. Removing vermin from the earth can in no way be a crime. God creates balance in the world; evil must be created to manage the good. Humans are purely neutral. They have a propensity toward evil, a little corruption can lead them down a path of evil viler than the depths of God's imagination.

Humans had an ability God could not possess, the ability to make the world better or worse. Humans are the moral arbiters of the world. While they play God's game, they are allowed to create their own rules and see how they play out. Heath believed if he was one of the rule makers, killing those that do evil was justifiable. Someone had to purge the world of the scum who brought evil into the world. Heath knew there were no good or evil people, but there were people who had so little good the deserved death. What could be more divine?

As Heath traveled he talked to people of all sorts. That was his favorite activity outside of the occasional begging. Socrates had taught him listening is one of the most important things one can do. Heath never liked twisting words and even retained a little resentment for Socrates when he had done so. Heath asked questions and listened. He asked farmers, merchants, bar girls, cobblers, soldiers, and everyone in between how they justified death. In Heath's search for vengeance, he encountered opinions of all varieties.

One said that since we are equal, violence is never justifiable.

One said that since we are equal, violence is only justifiable in self-defense.

One said that since we are equal, violence is justifiable to prevent future harm.

One said that since we are equal, violence is justifiable to get your way.

Yet another said violence is justifiable if it is to make the world right. And to him, Heath gave an ear. The man lived at home with his mother. Heath met him one day at a small bar. The place was similar to the one where Heath and Socrates met, perhaps that triggered something in Heath. A scraggly beard, unkempt man sauntered up to the bar with the confidence of a lion. He sat down and ordered a beer. Heath asked him his name.

"I am known to many as the man who figured out the world. The people here worship me."

"Oh?" Heath knew the man was lying. His weak frame couldn't be compensated by all the confidence in the world. His beady eyes seemed to look through everything, as if trying to see what he wanted, rather than what is.

"Indeed! I have written much, although I admit to sacrificing my physical health in this pursuit."

"And what have you written that has been so great?"

"Nothing you would have read, it probably would go over your head. But since you are so kind to pay for my drink I'll tell you."

"I'm not paying for your drink."

"Only a thief would declare an exchange of a drink for information as unfair."

Heath wanted to know how sick the man really was. "I'll pay. Tell me your ideas."

"Of course! I thank you for doing what you should, not many people do. Has it ever occurred to you that there is a beginning and end to everything?"

"No, because every end is a new beginning."

"A new beginning indeed! And one that shall never end."

"What's the point of this wordplay?"

"Then let me elaborate if you would only quiet your imbecilic mouth. I will attempt to lower my vocabulary for a brute such as yourself. I assume books have never been your fancy, your type never reads."

"My type?"

"Of course! I know you from your looks. I've seen your face on a thousand other mindless, dull bodies. After all, what are we other than what other people see as our groups?"

"I would prefer if you told me your whole ideas before assuming I agree with you."

"As you wish! I gladly tell anyone who listens, and even some that don't want to! Where shall I start? Well, let us go back to the beginning. Once upon a time we were a warlike people. We lived in the woods and constantly fought. Resources were scare, as we had no farms. We had to combat each other for the resources to win. Some time passed, and we realized that we could do much better in groups. We became attached to these groups. We started settling down and farming. This became the best way to live. People shared, and people prospered. But then a few people rose up and decided that they had the right to own what belonged to the group. These people are evil. They separated a unification of all people, and separated groups into sub groups, and sub groups into individuals. Do you see the problem? These individuals all belonged to groups. Some professed otherwise. How contradictory!"

"Time yet again passed and those who seized power rose to the top of society. They became our elected, our kings, our sovereigns. They made the rules by which everyone must live. In order to enforce those rules they made sure no outsider could enforce their own rules. And-"

Heath interrupted, "Are you implying there are not rules on which we all agree? Surely you believe we own something, if it as the very least ourselves."

"Typical of a brute, so selfish. Why would you own yourself? Why would you own anything? We are humans. We are a group. But we have divided that group. As humans, we each have the right to decide what is right, but we have no right to exert that upon other people."

"Yes, but that doesn't mean there aren't certain things we all agree upon which we can enforce upon ourselves. You have not killed me for my money, and I would not do the same to you. Any decent person would agree this is a rule."

"How dare you! How dare you assume you have the ability to decide what is decent and say that I must enforce your rules upon myself. I underestimated your stupidity."

Heath interjected again, "Sir, with all due respect, you are insane. I would propose a refutation, but that would be assuming your ideas do not refute themselves. However, I do enjoy listening to people and would like to ask you a single question. And no more nonsense, only answer this; When is it justifiable to use violence?"

"YOU AGAIN, START PUTTING THE BARRELS INTO PITCHERS. THE TOAST TO THRASYMACHUS WILL BEGIN SOON."

Without a moment of hesitation, Heath nodded and said, "Yes, sir." He didn't know Thrasymachus was the one being celebrated. He thought it was a military celebration. Heath should have known better. Why would the elite glorify their generals? War was useful, but its various practitioners should be kept at a distance. No need to trouble people and let them know the extent of the brutality by what can only be described as sadistic and perverted persons. The army had been known to make eunuchs of all their prisoners and use them as chattel.

Everyone seemed to act out in a controlling manner in this twisted society, and Heath would free them by ending the puppet masters. His hatred of Thrasymachus had enveloped his mind so much that he would not let anything stand in his way.

Heath's murderous intention was hidden behind his rugged and handsome face. He poured out two of the barrels into various pitchers until the cook came over and started helping.

"You're too slow."

"And you're not yelling?"

"I'm giving the lungs a break, and maybe my subordinates."

"Why?"

"Because I'm out of breath."

"No, why give the subordinates a break?"

"Steel can't be heated forever, it's got to cool. I hope my apprentices one day leave and surpass me, if they worship me after death I have failed. I want them to surpass me, but if I relentlessly demean they will never see me as anything more than a terrible teacher, one who believed in fear. Fear may inspire a few to excel, but why not challenge them all with love? I don't want a cabal of cooks from which only a few prodigies escape."

"You're smarter than your yelling makes you sound."

"POUR FASTER, WE STILL HAVE TWO MORE BARRELS."

Heath put the hood back over his head and reached down into his pocket. He fingered the coin Socrates had given to him so long ago. As he rolled it around in his hand, he walked through the servant door into the grand hall. Tapestries, statues, golden and silver ornaments, and every kind of gaud decorated the walls. Once he was done with the wine, the cook hadn't given two damns about where he went.

Heath took the servers door, sitting at a table of lower class men. They were the armed guard meant to protect the nobles and merchants. But who really cared? The town was safe, no army had been close in decades. Those meant to guard were drunk.

Heath sat on a stool a little off to the side. A few of the smarter men had similar positions. These were the men who had fought at war. They remained alert and didn't touch the alcohol. Heath had tried to figure out a way to assassinate them and failed miserably. It would have to come to a fight. If they paused for a moment to listen to him, perhaps he could persuade them to join. He didn't want a coup, just dead bastards. The sell swords would see that. Money was more important than loyalty. If they wished a coup, they'd be wealthy. Heath thought he could use this to turn them against one another, but it was a distant hope.

All Heath had to do was wait. He put his head down and fingered a piece of bread. The poison would act after about five minutes. At that point, the party would be in writhing convulsions. This would continue for another two minutes. Heath would stand up and announce the justice of the matter.

Heath went through the plan in his mind. He became lost in thought before he saw new flagons being brought out. They were a different color, servants whispered not to touch the glass until an announcement was made. Heath doubted the patience of many gathered.

After several minutes, a loud bell was rung several times by a servant. The man at the center of the table of a raised dais stood up. "Ladies and gentlemen! Thank you for coming to this great celebration of victory on the frontier. As Senate leader I am proud to announce our conquest of foreign lands is ever successful. While we can attribute this success to God, perhaps it is better to reflect on what we have done for the world.

We have brought water to the many. Through our genius engineering aqueducts carry water to lands so hot Hell recoils from them.

We have brought food to the hungry. These banquets are only possible because the farmers of the land and our scientists have worked together to create foods that last longer, effectively ending starvation in the winter.

We have brought law and order to the land! Order may have existed previously, but it was not lawful! A barbaric tribe may have enough order to exist, but not enough to exist as humans. Laws may have existed in some of these cities, but they did not promote order. These laws allowed elite classes to control subjects below them. Both situations are fit for savages! And we are not savages; we are the bringers of righteousness.

Today I propose a toast to celebrate our most recent victory on the front. Not only that, I would like to thank some of the benefactors who graciously contributed to this effort—namely, Thrasymachus. Through his ceaseless devotion to this country and donation of supplies to the army, our wars have been fought and won with great ease. My friend and fellow citizen, thank you for your work."

Thrasymachus waved his hand to applause. The Senate leader stood and raised his glass to drink. Heath smiled inwardly. He witnessed nearly everyone else down their glass. Heath took note of those who didn't.

The feast continued, with food being brought out on huge platters. Meats from foreign animals, vegetables from stolen land, all assortments of delectable accumulated on the tables. Heath didn't care. His hunger would be satiated soon enough.

In the back corner of the room, a man plummeted out of his seat and began clutching his chest. His face started turning a ghastly purple. The men around him thought he was making a joke. They laughed and ignored him. After another minute of clawing for air the man on the floor was joined by several others. The ruffians at the guard tables stood up and started shouting for help from the servants. Heath tried to contain his joy. A smirk worked his way onto his face, until he realized it would give him away. He shoved the smile back down into the recesses of his mind. There will be time for celebration later. The men, both the high and the low, started dropping like flies. In the chaos, Heath wormed his way to the dais at the opposite end of the room. He pushed his way over falling body, his sandals getting stained with vomit and piss along the way. Convulsions racked everyone who fell. It was as if each man had been struck by God for a sin they could never face. Heath could not help but contain his happiness.

The smile came back.

Heath reached the dais, coming up behind the row of bodies, some still moving, that made up the city's elite. He started with the living, cutting out each of their tongues with a rusty dagger he had bought earlier in the day. Blood spewed out of the mouth more than before, covering the marble floor. Heath worked his way to the middle, where the Senator lay dead and cold. Next to him, was the still gasping Thrasymachus.

Heath's hands were covered in gore. They dripped pure ecstasy. Heath sat on Thrasymachus' chest, preventing the dying man from squirming.

"Remember me?"

Thrasymachus was barely be breathing, his consciousness faded in and out. Heath came up with a brilliant idea. He tied the bag he was using to carry the tongues and tucked it in on his belt.

"Here, take this." Heath reached into a pocket and pulled out a vial. Quickly, he uncorked it and poured the contents down Thrasymachus' throat. Heath bent down next to Thrasymachus' ear, "You'll know what it is like to writhe in the justice of the divine."

Heath hadn't realized how easy it would be to get Thrasymachus out of the banquet hall. He encountered little resistance from the few men who restrained themselves from drinking. They were far too occupied with the situation at hand to take note of the bloodied man dragging a limp body out the server door. Heath pushed his way into the kitchen, leaving a red handprint on the decorative door designs. He was surprised to see it empty save a large figure over one of the myriad stoves.

"You know they'll blame me for this."

"I'm deeply sorry. There was no other way."

"I understand." Tears rolled down the head cook's face and onto the stove. They met the heat and evaporated into hissing puffs of steam.

"I thought you hated this…and them." Heath stated.

"I do, but I love my family more than the hatred. Without me, my kids will starve. My wife is weak and my daughters are far away. If they come back to find both parents dead, what would they think of us? Will they believe I killed everyone? I know that's what the bastards will say."

"They won't say a thing."

"Why?"

"It would mean they are vulnerable. It would mean they are weak. Any admission of these would be a unfortunate. You'll be taken care of silently if you choose to stay."

"I did nothing wrong. I choose to stay."

"That's a lie. You did something wrong. You worked at the behest of tyrants."

"I had no choice."

"No, you didn't like the alternative choices. You took the easy way out."

"Then I choose to accept my choice and stand firm, not taking the easy way out."

Heath paused for a moment. "Join me. I have a cart and we can settle in a village I know. It is far enough away no one will come for us, and close enough your daughters can visit if they choose."

The cook kept his face pointed downward. He told Heath his address. "If you show up, knock seven times on the door. If my wife or I answer, we will leave. If the response isn't immediate, we are dead or have chosen to stay."

"I'll be done in an hour."

Heath drug Thrasymachus' body outside the kitchen and into the unloading area. He threw the body into a barrel, closed the top, and put it into the cart. The stables were unsurprisingly empty of people. He opened the doors and drove off into the night.

Thrasymachus slowly opened his eyes and realized he was still alive. In a panic, he attempted to jump up, managing a pathetic arm spasm. A jolt of pain racked his throbbing head. He couldn't understand where he was.

Some kind of wooden cage. Fuck. I'm an idiot. I'm in a goddamn barrel.

"Help me this instance! Get me out of here!" Thrasymachus shouted, to no avail. He continued yelling until the barrel was promptly knocked over.

"Keep whining and we'll start a fire with the barrel."

Thrasymachus felt the barrel picked up and set straight. He could sense the bumpiness of the road in each rough bounce, but couldn't get a clue on the direction. The poison had left his body in a fugue-state, forcing Thrasymachus back to sleep.

"Get up, slime." Commanded Heath as he pushed the barrel over hard, knocking off the top. There was some moaning. The barrel rolled a few feet before Thrasymachus limped out.

"What do you want?" Pleaded Thrasymachus. His voice was weak and terrified. Thrasymachus could barely remember the events of the evening—everything had become a sickly fog of blood and pain.

"You're not asking questions." Heath kicked Thrasymachus. "Look at me, do you know who I am?" Heath grabbed Thrasymachus by his sweaty hair. It formed tangled knot in Heath's hands. "I said look at me, cunt." Heath punched the man in the jaw. Thrasymachus turned slightly and his eyes showed no recognition.

"I DON'T FUCKING KNOW." Heath was taken aback. The vengeance he wished to extract was for Socrates. How could he if the man didn't even remember Socrates? Heath thought before understanding the nature of his justice. "Good. I wouldn't want you to care about anything other than yourself." Heath drew his knife. "You aren't going to die tonight, I've changed my mind."

"Tha-thank you."

Heath smiled, "I took this idea from a good friend of mine, Robert. We were guards for a while together. Taking care of a merchant, Robert fell in love with his daughter. As per any relationship, the father was not happy. He had his own daughter killed and blamed on Robert. A singular daughter was of no consequence. The father had plenty of daughters with plenty of women. But the man wasn't done. He wanted Robert dead. But when news of his lover's death reached him, Robert went into hiding. One day, while the merchant was in town, Robert, disguised as a beggar, killed his two guards and drug the man into a valley near the town. And do you know what he did to him?"

"No."

Heath slapped him, "No SIR."

Thrasymachus whimpered, "Nnno sir."

"Better. Robert asked if the merchant remembered him. Of course, the man said yes. The proud captor asked the father if he wanted to live. Again, yes. Robert drew his blade, 'The world will know the monster you are. First, I shall remove your eyes. The beauty of the earth does not belong to one as evil as yourself. Next, I will take your right hand. For the theft you've committed you will be branded so all can see your nature. Finally, I will take your tongue. When you cry out in pain all that will emit will be a guttural screech. The world will not hear your prayers.'"

"Now, Thrasymachus my friend, do you know what I am going to do with you?"

"Please sir, don't."

"You're too quick to grovel. Who would have thought the sheep in lion's clothes would turn coward so quickly? What Robert did was merciful. Do you know where you are?"

Thrasymachus weakly looked around and whimpered, "No, sir."

"Of course not. Why would you know? Why would the great and mighty Thrasymachus ever visit a place like this? Do you see all these tied sticks? The crosses they form are there because they can't even afford to get an engraved stone. The city wouldn't dare give names to the poor. They are only "the poor" to you."

Heath sighed, "But, that's not why you're here. Do you see that stone?" Heath grabbed Thrasymachus' head and turned it slightly to the right. "Do you know who is buried there?"

Thrasymachus uttered, "No sir."

"I'm sure he'd have some arrogant retort if you hadn't butchered him." Heath took Thrasymachus and tied him to a nearby willow tree. The dirty creek that ran by the tree had turned its drooping leaves a sickly kind of yellow. Heath started, "This is for everything you've done, may it be long and painful."

"Wha-

Heath cut the man's chest. Not a deep slash, but enough to draw some droplets of blood. The next hour was spent disassembling the man piece by piece. Heath did his best to keep the man alive for all the more painful parts. Finally, the bloodied body started slumping. Heath grabbed Thrasymachus' face. "Wake up, here's the best part." Heath slapped the man, and Thrasymachus groaned. Heath drew out a dagger and began cutting right below Thrasymachus' breast. As he worked deeper, Heath slid a hand underneath the veins. He felt the organ pumping slowly. He looked Thrasymachus in the eye, "Fuck. You." Heath crushed his heart. Blood came flying out of the mouth, spraying the yellow leaves with darker red.

Heath went to the stream and pulled out a flask of water. He started rinsing his hands. Surprisingly, very little blood made it onto his clothing. He went back over to the cart and unhitched the horse. Hopping on, he headed off to the cook's house.

Heath knocked the required amount and waited. The street was one without night lamps, making it utterly dark. The sun had not yet begun to rise. Heath counted his lucky stars that there had been enough time to finish his long and tiresome quest. Now all that remained was escape with his newfound companion.

Heath stood there in the dim light and waited. He picked up a slight sound coming from behind him. Heath quickly turned and drew his sword. In front of him was a small woman, about a meter shorter than Heath. Heath remained calm, turned around, and slammed the door open. On the floor lie the cook, knife in hand. Heath took one look at the pathetic bastard. His eyes were wide with terror and his limbs trembled. "Please, I just wanted to save my family."

"I could have saved them."

"You can't even save yourself!"

Heath shook his head and turned away. "If you say anything to anyone about who I am I will know. I may one day perish. The ghost of my soul, however, will stalk you and yours for their cowardice for as long as your generations exhibit it."

Blast it all to hell, I thought I had something there. Heath disarmed the woman by grabbing her wrist. "And who are you?"

"Elizabeth, his daughter."

"Don't be an idiot and work around the wealthy. It always ends poorly." He let her go and walked out into the night.

Interlude 2

Hope: If that's not antithetical to everything I stand for I don't know what is.

Ramadi: You are the evil ones. You'd carry out an act for what?

Hope: Because you and your ilk are evil.

Chris: Who cares? We're good at telling stories. You're both wicked women in my view.

Triangle: Watch it.

Cortez: Keep the general's name out of your mouth.

Dmitri: Keyboard.

Cortez: What?

Dmitri: Keep the general's name off your keyboard. We aren't talking; we're online.

Ali: Dmitri's right.

Chris: This is one hell of a night. I'm glad the monastery finally finished brewing the wine.

Kant: Monks can drink alcohol?

Chris: Drink it? We make it! Someone has to taste test, and I put that burden upon myself. However, you get to reap the benefits of my cheerful attitude and charm that accompany a drunken state.

Ali: I will never understand this hedonist.

Doc: I'm up. Time to lighten the mood.

Mr. Anderson

Awakened by a pager, Charles sat up too quickly. His stomach lurched, his hangover struck like a hammer. An audible "Goddamnit!" escaped from his lips. *Why do they need me now? I'm supposed to get at least four hours. Fucking VA rotation is worse than surgery.* He reached over to his nightstand

and pulled out a bottle of over the counter painkillers, popping a small handful. Charles turned on the flickering bedroom light bulb. A bug experienced its last moments as the small body was rendered dead by the electricity. Early fly gets the fry, huh mate?

Charles took a terse ten minutes to get ready for work. The hospital expected a low modicum of cleanliness from students, and that provided Chris and excuse to let his self-care go to shit. While the slave like hours of residency drove many to the brink of insanity, the students often carried out their duties without a shower.

A few hours later Charles reached the old stone building in the middle of the city. He brought his bike inside; leaving it outside had cost him before. He learned every pile of mangled metal was attractive to thieves, if it had two wheels. Charles rested the cycle on the wall next to an assortment of others. You could tell which belong to whom by the shine. The doctors and nurses had high-end vehicles, but rarely bought new ones. They relied on something until it fell apart. It was the administrators that came in with a new set of wheels every month. The amorphous pile of resident bikes could have made a modern art piece.

Charles adjusted his dirty scrubs and walked down the hall to another locked door. The hospital had recently taken a liking to security. The building was full of veterans with afflictions ranging from degenerating bodies to decrepit senses, consequences of the poor bastards' trials by fire. Among all those who entered the building the one constant, a degradation of the mind, took place.

Charles walked past the nurse station and asked where he was needed. He was told to visit Mr. Anderson on the fourth floor. He would need another surgery today, but a lengthy explanation had to take place first. Goddamn bureaucracy. The old man doesn't care, let's just make it easy and load the clip for him.

Mr. Anderson was an enlisted army veteran. He served as a first lieutenant in one of the country's many wars abroad. He never specified which war, and the residents were told not to ask (Charles assumed it would induce a pernicious flashback). When the lieutenant returned from the war, Mr. Anderson's wife had left him for another man. His night terrors in the bedroom frightened his late spouse Elena. She viewed him as a killer, and as such, a father that should not raise children. His college age daughter, when she wasn't a hedonist, reviled him for his deeds. Her professors spoke with disdain for those who fought for imperialism. They infused the mind of a young woman with propaganda which changed depending on the decade. Academics had done this for years.

Mr. Anderson resided in a ceaseless drunken stupor. Depression was not the right word. His hospital caretakers had observed Mr. Anderson lacked the attributes of typical of a suicidal veteran. When engaging with doctors, Mr. Anderson would tell stories of valor. Often, he would insert himself as the hero in some ancient Greek or Norse myth. His attention would fade in and out, as if his own reality was blurred by his madness.

The man was admitted to the hospital last month after being discovered sleeping on the street covered in garbage bags. His military ID was still on him, which probably saved his miserable life. He was brought into the VA hospital and admitted to a room built for the rotting.

A quick examination of Mr. Anderson revealed he had a disgustingly yellow and red bandage wrapped around his right leg. Charles, who was working on his fifteenth hour that night, called for a doctor to unwrap the cloth. A wretched smell permeated the room once the wound was revealed. Medical students see a lot, they have iron stomachs. Seeing blood and guts and bones had to become a thing the mind filtered away. On that day, Charles experienced the only time an injury would make him sick. Charles, after unbounding the leg, retched when he saw two gangrenous toes that fell off the man's foot.

Since that day, Mr. Anderson had been treated for his mental state and the gangrene that continued to creep up his leg. Every so often, the VA surgeons would have to hack off another part of the limb to save the rest. Today would be the final surgery; the doctors had decided nothing below the knee could be saved. As he walked up to the fourth floor, Charles tried to piece together how exactly he could convey the unfortunate news. On one hand, Mr. Anderson would be unaware of what Charles was saying and try and tell one of his stories. On the other, by refusing to tell the man what was happening Charles legally accepted responsibility for Mr. Anderson's response.

Fucking A man, if only being a resident didn't include a VA or gynecology shift I life would be so much easier. Charles opened up the stairwell door and looked around at the whitewashed halls. The most divine colors are used to mask the most devilish of things. As he progressed down the hall, Charles noticed something odd smeared across the floor of the hospital. A yellow-red stain emitted a reeking smell that Charles' uncaffeinated mind had barely noticed. Residents learned quickly to block out smells and sights, but this was completely out of the ordinary. Charles picked up the pace and followed the trail. It had a strange pattern; it certainly wasn't human. Charles rounded the corner and realized he was right next to the floor's nurse station.

"Did you guys not see this?" A group of bleary-eyed scrubs looked up at him. Coffee did wonders for staying awake, but little to assist in cognitive function once the body reached a certain state of exhaustion.

"What the hell are you talking about?" Asked an older nurse.

"How the fu-" Charles realized the stain was below the counter of the station. Something small must have made its way past the station unnoticed.

"Never mind, I'll take care of it."

A muffled group of affirmative grunts came back in response. What the hell is going on? I better be dreaming or hallucinating. Charles tried to reason out exactly what was happening as he approached the stairs but came to no conclusion. I'm not tired enough to start hallucinating smells, am I? The stairwell on the opposite side of the hospital matched its drab sister. The slightly grayed steps circled their way up, protected by an iron guard. The smear struggled up the stairs, and Charles followed in intrigued anticipation.

The fifth floor held the recreational area. The pathetic floor for fun and exercise gave off the same stench of death as the rest of the building. The hospital was a funeral home for those waiting to die. At this time of night, the floor should have been closed off. However, that rarely stopped the permanent residents from going up.

Why are you convinced it's a resident? It could still just be a bloodied animal. Why is there an animal in the hospital? How would an animal make it all the way into the hospital, up the stairs, across the floor, and back up the other steps? It must be a person.

The automatic lights turned on when Charles entered the hallway. A chill raced down his spine. It was something straight out of a horror movie. You're being inane. The anxiety is definitely a part of your tiredness.

The smear continued down the hall and made an abrupt stop at the doorway of the computer lab. The residents weren't supposed to be able to access the desktops, let alone the room, this late at night.

Charles pushed open the unlocked door and saw a faint glow coming from a corner. The light ever so gently illuminated the face of a dead man. Charles' reaction of fear was taken over by morbid curiosity. He approached the chair in which the body slumped and saw it had a bloodied half leg as a limb. Charles looked at the computer, wondering what he had done in his final moments and read the lines

I am Mr. Anderson. I am Mr. Anderson. I am Mr. Anderson. I am Mr. Anderson. I am Mr. Anderson. I am Mr. Anderson. I am Mr. Anderson. I am Mr. Anderson. I am Mr. Anderson. I am Mr. Anderson. I am Mr. Anderson. I am…

Mr. Anderson would only be remembered by Charles and the children that he would tell about the first death of Mr. Anderson. He fulfilled Mr. Anderson's wish to a degree, passing on the universal tale of a fading life of glory, service, and pain.

Interlude 3

Hope: That was horrifying.

Divo: I've seen worse.

Dmitri: Divo, in what possible way have you seen worse?

Divo: Ever shovel manure?

Sumac: What kind of barbarian are you? How can you even use this machine?

Divo: Lots of practice.

Chris: I like Divo's life.

Divo: Why has this become a referendum on me?

Kant: Why not?

Dmitri: Shut up old-timer.

Kant: I'm only 50.

Dmitri: Old. Timer.

Hope: Mitri's right old-timer.

Ali: Don't worry old-timer, as Priest of State I'll issue your final rights.

Chris: Why do you flaunt your title?

Ali: Because I'm the Priest of State and you aren't.

Cortez: You're a fool.

Diog: Said the guy who volunteered for war.

Sumac: For heaven's sake let's stop talking about the labor of the poor. I'm up.

The Boulder of Sisyphus

It's not as though Nif was worse of compared to anywhere else. The rest of the world had long since fell to a nuclear holocaust. The previously extreme environments devoid of life became the last places hospitable regions. The remnants of civilization founded large cities and self-segregated. Isolationism became the only option. Fear of the fellow man was instilled through uranium and incompetence.

The giant city of Nif stood three hundred years against the storms of the desolated world. The same rulers who founded the city after the collapse still sat atop its hierarchy. How they managed to live so long kept a secret from the population. Massive stone walls surrounded a city that was the size of the long-decimated New York. The population, however, was kept at a severely regulated level. They needed people to work and reproduce just enough to keep a life of luxury for the rulers. Aleks wasn't sure these almost mythical creatures existed. They were never seen or talked about. The only hints to their existence were the Brutality Officers, the strange pyramid structure made of glass in the middle of the city, and the occasional announcement over the loudspeakers in the city. The Founders (they had a million different names) were responsible for the misery and suffering of an entire population.

One blasted day, a blizzard struck.

It provided the perfect opportunity to escape. The Brutality Police would be busy checking that the population didn't freeze to death in their brutalist homes. Aleks and Mika had been planning an escape for years, since they first met. Long hushed talks in a room where the only communication was through notes later burned carried their schemes to freedom. If someone heard them blaspheming against Nif, they would be reported and hauled off to fates that incurred far greater suffering. It was all too easy to be turned from a slave to subhuman chattel. Surprisingly, there was a difference.

Aleks finally reached his building currently being covered in snow. The architecture mimicked the brutalist structures of the old USSR. He was told they lived in an area that was once inhabited by the slaves of that regime. Aleks' namesake resembled the deceased Russians, his only connection to any sort of past. They taught him that much.

Education began at age 4 when the state transferred you from selected breeders to propaganda schools. These men and women were top specimen (as defined by the Founders). Kids were taught how they were lower than dirt, it was their kind which had destroyed the Old World. To their credit the schools, meant to disassociate the individual, taught about some sociocultural aspects of the Russians. Aleks thought this disconcerting, what was real and what wasn't? It seemed there was a group consensus among the population to just give up and accept what they were taught as fact. When you give someone a kernel of truth, it becomes significantly easier to wrap it in a coat of lies.

Morality didn't exist in Nif (hard to be good when everyone is equally bland). As such, the professors utilized the degraded society as part of the test was to see if children could survive on their own. They were taken at age 12 and sent to work in the thorium mines. The labor was specifically designed to kill just enough of the kids, while the survivors would be put into the populations. Those whom excelled beyond what was expected were placed into the breeder program. No better fate could come. Lives of relaxation and luxury, the breeders were pampered to no end. The whole system was orchestrated by the Brutality Officers, who allegedly got their commands from up on high.

Aleks couldn't stand it. Not knowing what things were true, who was in charge, or what was really going on set his psyche on edge. His whole life he fostered a desire to escape. He wasn't sure what it was, but something deep inside his soul yearned for freedom.

The young man understood why others felt differently. He had been shocked when he was young, one of his peers he discussed escaping with notified the authorities. Because Aleks was young, they only beat him for a short time. People prefer safety to freedom, even when that safety comes at the cost of human dignity.

At least Aleks had a small smidge of himself resembling dignity. Such a thing was impossible to find, and it was this small remnant of what once was that pushed Aleks towards Mika, and their plans for escape.

Aleks thought fondly of the woman. She had been his lover for several months now. They were permitted to engage in these affairs, the men and women had internal surgeries to prevent the production of kids. The primal act of sex was enough to keep the population in check. Devoid of most others pleasure, the carnal act accomplished the necessary human functions the fear and intimidation couldn't.

The night Aleks and Mika got together started off like any of the others, a dismal day of meaningless work followed by a night of nihilism. Aleks, arriving home from the job, saw the beautiful woman moving her small box of personal items into the building. She moved out of her old apartment because it was just time to do so. The rules and reasoning for these things were not known. Transfers were common, Aleks guessed because it prevented people from forming legitimate bonds with others. (It's not as though moving was difficult either, possessions were few and far between.) Friendships were banned by the Brutality Police. The only source of camaraderie was to be found in their acceptance as slaves.

That day Aleks and Mika slept together, expecting nothing more than the normal rush of endorphins received from the release. Afterwards, they stared at the gray ceiling, lying together in the uncomfortable bed made of metal covered with a stiff mattress. Mika had turned toward the window that faced one of Nif's walls outside. The structure was erected a mere ten steps from the concrete wall on the eastern side of the city.

She let out a sigh. A sigh. An emotive action. One beyond sex. Aleks knew, at that moment, he had to take a chance. The adrenaline rush would either see him dead, mindless, or free. Considering the outcomes of ignoring her cry for help, Aleks thought it would at least provide him with enough a story to think about the rest of his life.

He sat up and faced the black-haired woman. He didn't really look at his partners. A hole was a hole was a hole; the rest didn't matter. When Aleks opened his mouth to speak his tongue caught. For the first time in his life, he saw something beautiful. The woman next to him was utterly stunning. Her skin was a pale white, but not sickly. It shined like a source of innocent life in the midst of Nif's suffering. Her hair, not well kept, tried to shine despite the grime. It stood in stark defiance of all that blended together. The black stood out against the gray. Aleks fixed his mind and gathered up what was once called courage.

He put his hand gently on her shoulder.

"Mika?"

"Hm?" she turned back toward him, gazing into his eyes with the crystalline blue that made hers look deeper than any pit of depression.

"Why do you look like that at the wall?"

"Because I want to die."

"We all do, we keep on living despite that."

"Why?"

Aleks thought for a moment. He hadn't considered it. He was sure some people had killed themselves in Nif before. For some reason, he couldn't remember a single time where this had happen. Why did everyone keep choosing to live? Why did he choose to do so? Death would at the very least be an escape from this reality.

"Maybe they're scared what happens next is worse."

"What would that be?"

"I...don't know."

Mika took his hand off her shoulder. She sat up, facing him, those perfect eyes piercing a soul never touched.

"I want to die. It's pointless, like everything else. If I am going to die, I am going to make it meaningful." She emphasized the last word by folding her arms and furrowing her brow.

"Okay."

"That's it? You're like the rest of them. Unconscious and content to remain."

"I only said okay."

"You said it as a definitive."

"Mika, let us do something meaningful. I don't see why we have to die."

"What other meaningful thing could there be? Rebellion isn't an option, remember all the ones that failed?"

"They taught us, although it doesn't mean their reality is the only one. I have a better idea, one that's drawn me in since the day I saw the sun."

"You were outside that day?"

"No, I saw it through the window near my work station."

"Was it glorious?"

"I can't describe it." In reality what Aleks had seen was the simple shimmer of a small fraction of a ray from the dirtied glass of a factory. The sky above had long since turned gray, light no longer broke the surface.

"Are we going to do it?" Mika asked.

"Yes." Aleks said, lying through his teeth.

Aleks opened the door. The apartment building had eight floors, with twenty rooms on each. There was a communal kitchen and bathroom on each of them. A pretty standard building in Nif, this is what the majority of the population lived in. The temperature was kept well regulated, at a constant sixty-seven degrees. Air was pumped from somewhere down below. That was in fact the inspiration for Aleks' escape plan.

Getting around the walls would have been impossible. There was no way into the walls, and sure as hell no way to climb up them. Aleks couldn't remember ever seeing anyone perched atop the wall, he figured what was required to leave that way had been destroyed or lost.

With that said, the only way one could possibly hope to escape is through the underground. Aleks knew from working some stints that there was in fact an elaborate system. He had been on sewage maintenance, and worked to clear the large underground waterways of muck. While working, he noticed many roped off areas that were lit. They existed for some reason, and Aleks hoped they led to somewhere.

They would go on sewage shift the next day. It had taken a lot of time and proper arrangement for them to end up on the same shift. There were several sections of jobs one was assigned to. Ultimately the choice was p to the Brutality Police, but the people of the city were allowed to choose from the available sections. Specific roles within sections were assigned randomly, to prevent anyone from becoming too familiar with one skill.

It was the third time Aleks and Mika had signed up for the Cleaning section. The first two attempts they were assigned to one of the other jobs. Thankfully, the sewage clean ups tended to take in a lot of people. The workers would split into teams of five and skim the water with nets to get out any of the grime and dirt which fell from the sky every time it rained, and waste which occasionally accumulated.

Aleks and Mika were planning to overpower the other three in their group. Mika had even dared to suggest they should try to convince them. Aleks knew otherwise. He and Mika would knock them out and throw them in the sewage. If Aleks and Mika didn't kill them, the others might run back and report Aleks and Mika to the Brutality Police. (Reports on others always netted one a small score of flavored gruel.) By killing the others, Aleks and Mika could earn themselves another day. When the group didn't show up for their jobs the next day, there would be a search of their apartments. Aleks couldn't guess what would happen next. He estimated they would gain an extra day by killing. He just hoped he could go through with it.

Aleks made his way up to his floor and the room he shared with Mika. One was allowed to get a double sized room if they lived with a partner. It encouraged sex, which was a useful distraction from the overall malaise of depression. Opening the door, he saw Mika jump back a little, her blue pale blue eyes growing large in fear.

"Mika, it's just me." Aleks closed the door. Mika ran over and threw her arms around him.

"I'm so scared." She whispered into his chest.

What had happened? She was the stronger one. Mika was the leader who kept pushing for the escape, whenever Aleks would get nervous. Why was she upset now? He needed her to be strong.

"We'll get through this. I promise." Aleks regretted using the word. He had half done this in hope of death. If Mika and him were separated…He couldn't think about it.

"I know we will." She pulled back, wiping her eyes. "It was some dust. Don't think too much of it." She turned away and huffed. She was packing small satchels they had carefully made out of small pieces of cloth. They would attach the small pouches to the inside of their clothing. That was another benefit of the sewer crew; they had to wear several layers of clothing. No one was sure why, Aleks guessed it had something to do with the dust.

"I think we should have enough for two weeks." Mika said.

That was it; they had two weeks. Could they even get outside the sight of the walls if they walked for two weeks? Aleks' mind kept telling him to give up. That the months spent preparing, bringing back food to the room by stuffing it in his mouth, starving himself for days. The meal pills they were served tasted like grey, except on holidays celebrating the founders. Then the boring things tasted a little bit sweeter.

The gruel was packed with nutrients, enough to keep a person going for several days without anything else. There were a few kinds. One was packed with a lot of calories, another with the total worth of a normal day's calories and nutrients, and two others full of either fat or protein. Aleks and Mika had saved up a bunch of the high calorie pills, and had about half as many with fat or nutrients. The couple figured they would run as much as they could for the first week at least. They had been preparing themselves, choosing to do the cardio workouts in the morning. Every citizen was required to do a workout five days a week, to keep them in moderately decent shape. (It decreased stress and the likeliness of suicide as well.) A healthy population was more effective at their jobs. The Brutality Police didn't care who did what exercise. There were more than enough gym buildings scattered through Nif that no one exercise group was ever filled up.

"Let's rest up for tomorrow…and whatever happens next." Mika said. She was already in her nightclothes, which consisted of a gray cotton shirt and loose shorts. Aleks switched into his nighttime outfit, which was the exact same.

"We can do this." Aleks said, putting his arm around Mika. He pulled her close and kissed her cheek. They had felt strange about sex for a while. It was one of the things the Founders granted the people the freedom to find pleasure in. Abstinence was therefore an act of defiance, a refusal to adhere to the rules set up by those in power.

Mika turned out her lampshade, one of the few luxury items available in Nif.

Aleks put on the long overcoat carefully. He had to make sure when he moved the pouches out of his bag and into the coat no one noticed. Mika came over and stood in front of Aleks. It was normal to engage in small talk conversation. It showed you weren't going insane. Any sign of mental illness and the Brutality Police sent you to become chattel.

Aleks took advantage of Mika's positioning, and quickly shoved all their gear into both of their pockets. It took him five seconds, just enough time for a thorough conversation. Anyone watching wouldn't be able to tell what was really happening.

"Now for the fun." Mika told him, her eyes smiling. She was actually enjoying the whole experience. Real, true joy. That, or her adrenaline was running so high she no longer had a concept of cowardice.

Either way this all depends on our partners. Aleks hoped it was three women. Women rarely participated in weight training as much as men. And the men who willingly opted for sewer duty tended to be stronger and meaner than the rest. Thankfully, women dominated this job, because it was paired with several indoor cleaning jobs under the Cleaning section of work. The odds were you'd end up in one of the nice jobs inside, maybe by yourself. Times where you were alone were priceless.

Aleks followed Mika out of the changing room and into a hall big enough to fit one hundred people. A member of the Brutality Police stood atop a raised dais at the back of the room. Gradually, more people filled the room. The Brutality Officer pulled out a sheet of paper and began to read off names. The Officer had decided that some people needed to be separated. When twenty people (mostly men) were called and put into special groups overseen by Brutality Officers, the rest of the workers were told to form groups of five. There were more than enough women, so Mika and Aleks grabbed three without arousing any suspicion.

The first woman was short and squat. Her broad shoulders looked like they could carry a heavy weight, although she barely reached up to Mika's shoulder. The second girl had a similar complexion to Mika (slightly lighter hair and a fatter nose). The last girl looked like she was ready to fight at a moment's notice. The citizen's in Nif had most of their emotion trained or beaten out of them, yet this woman had a fire lurking behind her eye. Every movement she made was purposeful, as if she were a member of the Brutality Police with a citizen to go beat up. The woman was about Alek's height, had long legs, and a busty chest the large, protective overcoat couldn't hide.

We might have a chance with them. Aleks thought, believing that they could at least convince the fire-eyed woman.

"Embark, now." The Brutality Officer announced from the stage. The groups went up to him to receive their maps. The groups were supposed to follow the designated route on the map, dredging up anything in the water that looked to be a contaminant. They were supposed to pour iodine powder into the water as they walked. The routes ended up circling back to the big room, where the citizen would tun in their gear. Aleks and Mika had studied the map religiously. The chances of running into another group were slim to none because the underground sewer was enormous. It was continually expanded each day, the rumblings felt throughout the whole of the city. Aleks had discovered where one of the work sites was. He hoped they could find a way out from there. There had to be an escape to the sewers outside the city, his intuition told him. No one would construct this fortress without a way for a spy to escape the ire of his peers. Aleks knew there were plenty of the cowards scattered throughout the city. They were a branch of the Brutality Police called "the Pigeons." The Pigeons acted as normal citizens, but disappeared sometimes to make a report on their neighbors who may be trying to engage in illicit activity. The underground market for alcohol trade was the biggest issue (the punishment for which was being turned into chattel). The Pigeons kept everyone on their toes, fearing the repercussions from talking with one to many people.

Aleks' group went up to the officer to receive the map. The officer who handed Aleks the parchment lacked any emotion on his face. The stone from which he was chiseled weathered more change than the tightly pulled lips and stern eyes of the officer. The Brutality Police were a different breed of human. They stood over six feet tall, with short buzzcuts. They, like the rest of the citizens in Nif, were forbidden from growing out their facial hair. They were supposed to be hulking masses of interchangeable units. The Brutality Police had eyes which were a dark brown, their skin a few shades darker than the average population. Muscles corded their bodies, no citizen could begin to consider reaching the same level of fitness. Aleks had guessed they were fed some sort of drug to make them that way. He drew the conclusion from the fact he never saw the same officer more than two years apart. The drug likely made them stronger, but destroyed their lifespans.

The group continued forward into the cave, accompanied by three other small groups, for five minutes before reaching the first major branch. The giant tunnel separated into twenty-one diverging paths. Some led straight down to the lower sewers, while others climbed a little. Only three of the paths stayed on the same level of sewer.

Aleks had estimated form his past work in the sewers there must be some thirty levels to the sewer. How they managed to build so far down, he had no idea. He thought the rock would be too hard to get through, however the city seemed to have found a way. Aleks thought it likely the previous Founders had used technology long lost to construct these waterways. The new Founders kept up the construction as a ruse to demonstrate they still maintained scientific and industrial dominance.

He hadn't brought most of his theories to Mika, fearing she would think him crazy. This was one he did bring up, as it was crucial to the escape. They did their best to memorize the layout, however there were so many branching avenues (some of which weren't listed) it was nearly impossible. Mika's mind was much sharper than Aleks, so she was the one who laid out and memorized their specific route. Aleks felt somewhat useless. Something in his bones he had a responsibility to take care of her. It wasn't love that drove this feeling, it was the innate desire to protect a woman. Aleks had this feeling some times before, watching women be dragged away by the Police. Aleks just hoped he wouldn't have to do anything horrible to the women with him.

Aleks, Mika, and the others in their group walked forward silently on one of the paths which went downwards at a sharp angle. Water rushed by, and the team began to set up their equipment. Two members would be on one side. The first pulled the large net, which spanned the length of the channel. The other would slowly dump iodine from a pump attached to their backpack into the water every forty steps. The same was mirrored on the other side, except one of the team members (this time it was Mika) carried a net with smaller mesh, to fish out anything that may have escaped.

Aleks and Mika were on opposite sides, Mika having the squat girl and the fighter. Aleks walked behind the other woman.

The woman who looked like Mika introduced herself to Aleks as Katarina. A common name. Aleks lied and told her his name was Lantis, another ubiquitous name in Nif.

It was normal for the sewer groups to make small talk. There wasn't much to discuss, they all lived similar enough lives. The most frequent topic of conversation was sex, as it was the only variety anyone had.

The conversation went that way for some time, each talking about the different people they had slept with. Aleks intentionally left out anything about Mika, scared Katarina might spook.

Through a series of twisted tunnels, Aleks estimated they were three or four levels down. Luckily, he was the only one with the map, and started to take ques from Mika. She would make small signals with her hand as to where to go. When Katarina asked if Aleks if he knew where he was going, he gave a curt nod. It was best to seem mildly depressed and annoyed at all times.

After an hour and a half (Aleks counted his breaths to measure time) Mika stopped suddenly. She stood behind the two on her side. The group turned toward her, the squat girl asked, "What's wrong?"

Mika, without skipping a beat, replied, "We're escaping."

In that moment of silence, a million seconds passed. Aleks and Mika could be turned into murders if a single one of them refused. Katarina was the one to speak up.

"About time."

"What?" Aleks was gloriously surprised by her response.

"We're escaping. We planned this from the beginning. The other two over there are in with me. We've been saving supplies and had planned on leaving when we had enough."

The squat woman continued explaining, "We can't stand it. There's nothing to do besides sex. We should do something interesting, and I'm not keen on getting arrested. Which means the only thing left is escaped."

The fighter turned to Mika, "Do you know how we're escaping?"

"I have a rough idea."

"Michelle worked for the engineering groups the past few years as much as she could. She learned the layout of the sewers and discovered some irregularities."

Aleks listened intently, acutely aware of how their conspiracy echoed through the tunnels. One couldn't make a sound in the sewers without it being heard a hundred steps away.

The squat girl, Michelle, smiled—her once stern face lit up. "Are you ready for an adventure? I think I found an escape. Katarina, come over here."

Aleks and Katarina backtracked two minutes before finding a bridge. They were set apart every ten minutes. Walking back to the group Aleks felt he needed to make up for his lie. Another deep belief within his unconscious mind said lying was wrong. Like the protection for women, this innate feeling couldn't be described or articulated.

"My name's really Aleks." He said, a small bit of red rising to his cheeks.

"I figured you lied. You were suspicious from the start." She said, smiling. "Thank you for telling me."

When they reached the others, Michelle, Mika, and the other girl discussed how they would met out the supplies between them. Aleks and Mika had run some tests in the apartment, and found one could go a week and a half without food and still be functional. Water was a different story. If they found a way out of the sewers, they would need to acquire supply and a way to carry it more efficiently. The small water bottles they had wouldn't be near enough.

The fighter, Catherine, had started getting jumpy. "It's time we get moving. The bigger the head start, the higher the chance of survival."

"Aleks, Michelle, take us out of here." Mika said. The group quickly dropped the cleaning supplies into the sewer and continued on.

The mood was strangely uplifting. Everyone was excited. The adrenaline spike would wear off, but man was the rush good. Aleks brought his lips to an unconscious smile.

"What's that for?" Michelle asked.

"Its thrilling. We're going to escape."

"How can you be so sure?" Michelle showed the least emotion of anyone. Her face read like Brutality Officer, her stern gaze boring into one's skull.

"I…don't know but that's better than the alternative!"

"You're strange."

"You're escaping with me so I can't be that strange."

"I work with what I got." Michelle's face twitched in reaction to her internal happiness.

It was good to be with those who understood. They were united against a common enemy. That was all they truly needed. Aleks wondered if everyone in the city had felt the rumblings down deep in their bones. Was escaping the right option? Couldn't they help those back in Nif? It may have been a prison, yet even prisons can be homes.

They began to work their way further and further downward. The stonework grew older and less well kept. Moss and lichen grew in places where it should have been scraped off.

"We're not going to a construction site?"

"How would that help us?" Michelle huffed. She hated unnecessary questions.

"I thought that's how we could leave."

"What makes you think you would be able to leave from a place where they are digging new parts of the sewer? Are you stupid?" Michelle snorted, "Dumb question. The weird irregularities appeared on the lowest of the levels. My guess is they are so old they don't know what's down there anymore, and are too scared to investigate."

"Scared? Michelle, why would they be scared?" Aleks' joy faded a little and he felt the adrenaline more thoroughly course through his veins. He had to watch it, too much could make him irrational. In school they taught people to control their breathing and soothe their emotions. A docile population, including a dissatisfied and abused one, is easy to control.

"I found a reference to several deaths at those levels in recent years. Whenever a crew was assigned for clean up, they didn't return, save for one guy who came back stark raving mad."

"Stark raving?"

"Vocabulary hard for you? I guess you never worked in any of the more scholarly crews."

"You make too many guesses."

"Don't tell me what I do and don't do." Aleks had expected that kind of response from Catherine. He couldn't imagine what conversations between those two would be like.

The five carried onwards for another several hours, descending deeper and deeper into the caves. They had no way to keep time, and the steps dragged on. The citizens of Nif had been trained since birth to go to bed and awake at a certain time. It was one of the few biological engineering feats the Founders accomplished. This meant the entire group knew approximately what time it was. They had a chance of making more headway before anyone noticed. They may have the entire night. Come next morning, they would certainly be hunted.

"We should walk through the night." Catherine said. She hadn't a look of tired on her face. The fluorescent lights that adorned the sewer walls illuminated her eyes, highlighting her confidence. She wanted to escape far more than the rest. Aleks could sense it on her.

"I agree. Let's stop in another few hours. Hopefully they think we just got lost and follow the route we were supposed to take." Mika said.

"There's a lot of hope in you people." Michelle said. She was commending the group, her tone only made it seem like a condemnation.

"We have the supplies to survive. We just have to get to the black site." Aleks stated confidently.

"The black site? Is that what we're calling it now?" Katarina laughed at the name. "Works for me."

"The rest of you okay with that?" Aleks asked.

He was the most jovial of the group. Despite their femininity, each carried herself proudly—as if there were anything to be proud of. They lived under dictates they had no say in, with no way to escape, and when they tried they would likely end up dead. Their entire lives were spent doing labor they didn't know the purpose of, occasionally being able to forget all the toils thanks to some alcohol. They seemed put together from their gaits, every step echoing a variety of confidences. Meanwhile Aleks couldn't find the right words to articulate the way he felt, stumbling over his feet now and then.

"I don't see why we're bothering with talking. Save our breath, let's keep moving." Michelle stated, pointing down one of the branching corridors. "We only have a few more levels to go before we reach the site."

"It was that close?" Katarina asked, sounding surprised.

"There are more than one, there are ten I can see on this particular map. We got a lucky starting branch, that's all."

"Does anyone have a light? The ones on the walls might go out. It is a black site after all." Katarina stated. She had some sense of humor, unlike the rest.

"Shut up." Catherine said. "Let's keep moving."

Another two hours passed uneventfully. The lights on the walls seemed to fade slightly the more they traveled. Their spacing on the wall was also at a greater distance, sometimes forcing the group to walk in growing darkness.

"I don't like the water, it seems different." Mika said.

She pointed to the channel. It had turned a slightly different color. The dark blue was no marred my streaks of brown and grey, emitting a gross odor. Every now and then, Aleks thought he could see the surface being broken. Nothing save fear and anticipation came from the murky depths.

"We should watch out. I'd guess whatever killed those guys has to do with the water. I've never seen anything like this, and I've been in the sewers quite a bit." Aleks said, trying to squelch the fear in his voice. How are they so damn put together? I'm shaking.

"Catherine will kill it." Michelle stated, as if it were only a matter of fact.

"Cat" Katarina said, then apologized with a nod after noticing Catherine's response, "Catherine, can you take it?"

"How am I supposed to know what I can or can't take when I don't even know what the damn thing is! I'm not just hired muscle."

"What's that?" Mika asked. Aleks and Katarina shared a laugh; Michelle gave one of her snorts that seemed to indicate a mild form of amusement, or whatever Michelle's equivalent was. For the citizens of Nif, she was still rather stoic.

Mika handed Catherine the large fishing net. It was much of a weapon, but it had metal. It would be a good bludgeon, if anything else.

"Here's to fighting sewer monsters." Catherine said, hoisting the net above her head.

"At least they aren't rats. I always hated rats." Mika said. She seemed small compared to these three women. Aleks loved her deeply, but wondered how such a mouse had survived the harsh population controls. People weren't supposed to be this docile. Aleks adored that part of her. She was something precious to protect in this world. That's why he screamed when something leapt out of the water at his lover.

"WHAT THE FUCK?" Aleks yelled.

A scaled creature the size of a head broke the surface. It jumped at Mika, landing on the walkway. It was fat and bloated, about the size of two fists. Small teeth jutted out from the thing's twisted mouth at strange angles. As it flopped about on the deck, the group was shocked.

"What is that thing?" Mika gasped. She was more curious than terrified.

"I think it's a fish. Better throw it back, I don't know what to do with it." Katarina said. "I think we don't want to eat that. Something looks wrong with it." Catherine pushed the thing back into the water with the net, where it quickly swam away.

"Why did it jump out like that?"

"You must smell like food. You been eating shit recently?" Michelle asked the group.

"Only the same as you!" Katarina said laughing kindly. She didn't have a shred of fear in her body. Only curiosity pumped through her veins. Aleks knew why. As soon as one considered the consequences, the horrible fate that awaited them when caught, all that was left to do was sit and revel in the few brief moments of freedom they had left. The sheer, overwhelming fear of not knowing the unimaginable suffering that was bound to come would move an army of Atlases. Anxiety is too small a word to encompass the emotion that embraced the brain if one grew too lax. Laughing was the nicest of cures, something not frequently seen in Nif.

The group continued walking down the sewer. Strangely enough, the sewer started to angle downwards, and the water started to pick up speed. Michelle held up her hand to stop the group.

"Does anyone hear that?" She asked, turning back toward everyone. Aleks and the rest shook their head.

"Something's coming up ahead. It sounds like crashing of some sort. Constant, repeated crashing." She seemed concerned. "I think I know what comes next."

They continued for another hour, the noise getting louder and louder. It echoed down the hall, reverberating off the walls, occasionally causing small ripples in the water. Finally, the group spotted a large opening at the end of the tunnel. Water rushed over the side of the edge, disappearing into nothing. They were too far back to see over it.

"I think this is where we get killed." Katarina said. "A better fate than if we stayed back in Nif."

"It sounds pretty, I like it." Mika said, her warm smiled easing Alek's mind.

They continued forward cautiously. Every now and again, Aleks would look at the water, trying to spot the creature that attacked. It had to drag one of them into the water to kill. It was not too difficult a task, causing Aleks to glance at the fast moving water (which now looked more like slime.)

"Does anyone smell that?" Michelle said.

"Michelle, what kind of weird ability do you have? No one senses things before you." Aleks asked, genuinely amazed.

"I pay attention." She flicked a glance towards Mika and Katarina, who were joking about what they could possibly find.

"Maybe I can take a bath!" Mika said.

"Cleaning yourself is an important aspect of self-care." Katarina replied.

The group marched forward. The light from the opening of the tunnel was stronger than in the sewer currently. When the group reached the edge of the tunnel, they stood in amazement.

Light flooded in from far above. A giant ball of orang-yellow fire set deep in a pristine blue sky sent shimmering beams of light deep down into an unimaginably cavernous pit. Into this pit, flowed the contents of several sewer openings. Huge waterfalls of disgusting water marred with sludge and trash poured over the edge into the basin below. Around the bottom of the massive lake, there were small shacks made of miscellaneous materials. Small humanoid forms moved about, unaffected by the stench, light, or sound. The light, reflecting off the lake, next to people, free people, put a tear in Catherine's eye.

It was the most beautiful thing she had ever seen.

"I hate to ruin the moment, but how are we getting down? Do we want to go down, isn't up the correct choice?" Michelle asked.

"If those people got down they can certainly get back up." Katarina said.

"That's idiotic, who's to say they didn't fall and stay there?" Mika stated.

"We could ask them you know…" Aleks said. He was standing at the front of the group and realized what that meant. "Fine, I'll ask them."

Aleks drew in a deep breath and yelled down into the pit, "HELLO! WE'RE FROM NIF." His voice echoing down into the pit enhanced it ten times. The humans looked up to the ledges, spotting Aleks and Michelle waving furiously. They started to run into their shacks, carrying out some kind of large sticks. Aleks realized his mistake when they shook the sticks at the sewer exit.

"WE AREN'T POLICE, LOOK AT US!" Aleks shouted. The humanoids conversed some before a larger man began shouting back.

"HOW DO WE KNOW WHAT YOU REALLY ARE?"

Aleks looked around. That was a question Michelle should be able to answer. Instead, she deferred to him as the appointed liaison.

"YOU DON'T, BUT UH WE HAVE FOOD!"

The humans at the basin's edge talked for some more time before replying, "OKAY. WE ACCEPT. LOOK AT THE WALL TO YOUR LEFT."

That was fast. Aleks thought.

The man paused to draw a breath. Before he began again, Catherine had spotted the stone that was ever so slightly misaligned with the rest of the wall. She pressed the stone inwards until it clicked. Behind the wall the group heard a grinding sound.

"They use this a lot. Listen to the sound. If it wasn't used it would be all creaky." Michelle said.

An entire section of wall, stretching back twenty feet slid downwards into the ground. In front of them was a large stone staircase, lit by fluorescent lights set into the wall behind some glass. The staircase did a ninety degree turn about what Aleks estimated was halfway down, hiding the rest of the descent from the view.

Aleks shouted back, "WE FOUND IT, WE'LL BE DOWN SOON." With that the group started the walk down into the basin.

It took approximately an hour to reach the bottom of the steps. In front of them was a large door made of shiny metal. There wasn't a latch to open in. Aleks knocked on the door.

A window at Michelle's height opened up, with a pair of eyes peering at them curiously. There was a mix of fear and amazement in those young pupils. The child was moved aside, and a face of a much older man appeared.

"What is your business in Blight?"

Michelle snorted. "That's one kind of name."

Catherine stared the man dead in the eye. "We want in. We want out of Nif and safety."

The man nodded and closed the slit. A large object was hefted onto the ground, and the iron door pulled open by a group of young men. They looked less deformed up close. Aleks noticed the major difference in body type from his own. The men of Blight were corded with muscles that looked unlike the bulk put on by the Brutality Police. They were short but strong, with longish brown hair. Their eyes were universally brown or hazel, much different than the Nif citizens. Aleks smiled.

"You aren't from Nif, how'd you end up here?"

The old man who opened the slit looked at Aleks with some disdain, "We invite you into our home and the first thing you do is demand answers. We should eat first, follow me." The old man turned and led the to a shack placed against the pit's circular wall. The shack had a roof made of tin, upon closer inspection tin that was well kept. The old man pushed aside the cloth door, revealing a sand floor with a table and chair. There were some miscellaneous items necessary for a poor man's survival strewn about. The old man walked to the back of the wall.

"Watch this, kids."

He pushed on a stone in the same way as the one above.

"No way we could live in there with the water. It smells and is way too loud. We have long since pretended to be out there during the day, in case one of the city's police forces come by."

"Police forces? Plural?" Catherine asked, squinting.

"Relax, we won't have to fight. They don't know how to get down here."

"You didn't answer the question." She said, almost growling.

"How about you have some tea to calm down first?"

"Telling me to relax and calm down really isn't causing either to happen. What the fuck is going on here old man?"

The group audibly gasped. Swear words could get you in trouble with the Brutality Police. Aleks got away with it earlier due to the shock of the situation. But Catherine's words were out of anger. Anything outside the prescribed set of words and meanings was heretical. Although, Aleks guessed, it might be good to start using them. Just a "fuck you" to Nif.

"Tea first. I'll listen to your whining later."

The old mad led them down a small stone hallway into a giant antechamber. The hole was as big as Nif itself. Buildings rose up, carved entirely out of stone. The ceiling rose high (but didn't open up to the sun like Blight had) above their heads, decorated with beautiful works of art.

The tunnel let them out at a catwalk set near the top of the dome. Which meant the city had been built even lower than the sewers. Michelle's mouth was nearly watering as she spat out question after question.

"How did you manage to do this? Didn't you strike bedrock? Nothing can get through bedrock. And light? Why is it bright in here? Where do you get the energy to fuel the city? And where…" Michelle's eyes widened as she looked out over the city and saw cars.

"You have automobiles? And..you have a LOT of them!"

The old man turned back to Mika, a grin on his wizened face. "Welcome to Tartarus." He spread out his arms. Aleks didn't take note previous, but the city was much larger than he initially realized. He could barely glimpse the other edge.

The old man pushed another stone into the wall. This one wasn't hidden, it was marked out from the rest of the cobalt colored wall with an off white that had been worn by thousands of hands. A doorway into the wall opened, revealing a bustling chamber of people moving about. In the middle of the room were three pairs of tracks. One went down, one went around the catwalk, and the other disappeared upwards.

Catherine put a hand on the old man's shoulder. "We want to go outside. Let us go up."

"No. Its dangerous outside still. We must wait another ten years."

"WHAT? Ten years?" Catherine grew irate. The closer she drew to freedom the closer she felt it would be taken away. "We aren't waiting that long. Let us up."

"Fine, suit yourself." The old man led them to the track that went upwards.

"Wait, uh…what was your name?" Katarina asked.

"Ligmey."

"That's an unfortunate name." Mika whispered to Aleks.

"Ok Ligmey, what happened to the person who came back to Nif. Why was he crazy?"

"He broke when he saw Tartarus. It shattered his mind to know how close he was to our wonderful city, when he lived in Nif."

"I don't trust you, however, that answer works for now. Let's go." The strange resolute stoniness more prevalent in Michelle and Catherine's demeanor appeared in her tone. No wonder they ended up together.

Ligmey led them around to the train which headed upwards. The platform by it was distinctly less busy than the others.

"We should be one of the few going up, maybe some researchers." Ligmey told them. He and Michelle talked about how the train worked. They had a few in Nif that were mainly used for carrying large cargo in and out of mines.

The train sounded a horn and began to slowly chug its way upward. Aleks and Mika sat next to each other in one of the plush seats. The train was made so people sat in small, plush booths that could fit eight. The walls of the train were made almost entirely of glass, although each individual booth could pull down a curtain around their table. The roof was decorated in a mosaic depicting things with weird legs and hair, poking out all around. Aleks saw there were a few things that looked like the Nifian pigeons that populated the city.

The journey was mostly dark for some time; they had to climb for a long time to get this low into the bowels of the earth. The walls were carved of the same cobalt color as the ones of the city's rock walls. The stone faintly glowed, giving off an eerie light.

Catherine stared longingly out of the window. She had calmed down some, although her jaw was still locked tight. Katarina and Mika were joking with each other about the strange creatures on the ceiling.

Where is the light coming from? I don't see anything.

"Hey Ligmey, how can we see? There aren't any lights."

"The bluestone." He replied. Cobalt sounds much better.

"It looks too faint to have effect."

"That's because it's lighting the entire car. Put a bunch of little things together they sometimes make the whole picture clearer. We're coming to the exit now, prepare yourselves."

The train chugged along, its engine providing a comforting noise. Suddenly, the entire car was bathed in a blinding light.

"I KNEW IT! WHAT DID YOU DO!" Catherine shouted, hopping over the back of the booth then jumping into the aisle. "I CAN'T SEE!"

"Relax. It's just the sun. Look, there's no one here to harm you child." Ligmey said. He was surprisingly tolerant of Catherine's outbursts.

"Oh my goodness…" It was green. Brilliant, beautiful, green. They had only seen a variation of the color in its most sickly form of moss growing in unwashed toilets. Green covered the ground up until a large mountain range. Mountains so high they boggled the mind. Their peaks broke the clouds, and when they were seen they were covered in white powder. Not the ash that continually covered Nif, but a pure white. Mountains off in the opposite directions had a bluish tinge. The train pulled to a stop close to the exit.

"We aren't getting to see more?" Mika asked, her breath barely staying with her.

"You will. We have to stop here, there aren't any settlements beyond this exit which can sustain consistent life. The researchers here work, have been working, nonstop for a solution. We have plenty of photos and observation points, don't worry."

The train entered through a doorway made of bluestone. It shut behind the train without a sound. The locomotive pulled to a stop at a platform far smaller than the one they had left from. Not a single person stood waiting on it. When the train stopped, about a dozen men wearing blue pants and white shirts walked out. The majority wore glasses. The rest of their details were a wide hodgepodge. There were men with dark skin and poofy black hair, shorter men with eyes that looked squinted, men with tan skin and thick black eyebrows, and the tallest of them all, a man with pale skin and golden-brown eyes.

Aleks was amazed at their makeup. He pointed to the group and asked the old man, "What did you do to them?"

The old man started laughing. "What did we do to them? Well, we have fewer of the darker skinned fellows now that we aren't exposed to the sun as often. Other than that, I'm afraid you'd have to ask their parents. They are normal humans like you and I."

"But what about the people back in Blight? They looked…different."

"Short? You mean they're short?" The old man was having a grand old time of it, while the rest of the group looked around in amazement or listened with a look of confusion on their face. Michelle was smaller than the rest of them, but only by a few inches. They had never seen people as short as those in Blight.

"They are just shorter people, sometimes they come out like that."

"And the deformities?"

"Now that is a far more interesting question. We induce temporary deformities and fix them when the guards come off duty."

"They were guards?" Catherine asked. "I could have taken any of them."

"I'm sure you could have young lady. Enough talking, let's go to a more comfortable place." They followed Ligmey through a small corridor, which ended in a large glass dome. They could see in all directions from the dome. People bustled about their business, fewer than one hundred in totality. They carried a miscellaneous grouping of the characteristics more diverse than the group they originally saw.

The dome had several exits, all with glass doors that closed when someone wasn't using one. It was technology so far advanced it didn't exist in the minds of Nifians. It wasn't unrealistic—it was alien.

"This is amazing." Mika said, hugging his arm close to her. Aleks squeezed it. Being able to show affection publicly was not something he was used to. He felt a small warmth inside and kissed her on the forehead.

"Enough of that lovebirds, we have exploring to do!" Katrina said, practically bouncing up and down.

"Over here, I'll give you the tour later." Ligmey said. He brought them to a covered hub where people were sitting and eating.

"Where's the line?" Michelle asked.

"There is no line. You ask what you want, take a number, and when they call the number you pick it up."

"Anarchy." Michelle said disapprovingly.

"Would that be a bad thing?"

"We're told it is from the time were kids, but what do we know?"

"Astute observation. Here, take a seat first." Ligmey sat them down at a round table. While Catherine and Katarina were gawking at the scenery,

Michelle berated Ligmey with more and more questions.

"Do those three get hungry?" Mika asked.

"I don't know. Nif messed up making them." Aleks said.

"I kind of like them."

They looked at the giant light up menu in awe. "I don't know what most of these things are." Mika's confusion was warranted. The language was the same used in Nif, but the menu contained a variety of things they had never heard of.

What's a burger?

"Let's ask." Aleks walked up to the counter, there were several men standing there at different stations. Each wore a funny little hat and a smile plastered on their face. "Hi, we're new here. What can we eat?"

"What can you eat? Sir, you can eat anything on the menu if you can afford it."

"Afford?"

"Yes, afford it." Ligmey noticed what was going on and patted Michelle's hands. He hurried over and gave the boy a shiny black card. "Put my whole group on that."

"Yes, sir."

Ligmey looked at them, "I recommend getting the scalloped potatoes to start off, we can go from there. Your heritage is Russian, you should like this kind of meal."

The man behind the counter snorted. "Should we give them vodka and communism as well?"

Ligmey gave him a blank stare. "They are new, be kind to these people. You were once like them."

The man rolled his eyes. "Whatever. I'll put your order in."

The group went back to the table. Ligmey pulled Katarina and Catherine from their observation to the table. A waiter brought over a tray of tea and water.

"How much will this cost?" Aleks asked, only half joking.

"These are complimentary. Everyone drinks tea, and I imagine you five are starved for water. Let me explain what's going on briefly. If you have any questions," he said nodded toward Michelle, "I can show you to someone better suited to knowing our history. I'm just a guide for folks like yourself."

"Tartarus is one of two republican cities to make it through the wars. The earth was destroyed several times over by man's incompetence. Rulers thought they knew better than the people they ruled, so they attempted to enslave the underclasses with promises of free things. Nothing is free. Absolutely nothing. When it comes to services, someone has to provide them. When the population realized they would be the ones serving their higher overlords, they began to revolt. Most areas were squashed immediately. Europe was decimated by wars which descended into vulgar tribalism. Africa was drained of resources and enslaved for labor. East Asia sided with either China or Japan. America became more and more divided and totalitarian. Of all the places in the world, the only cities with republican interests that survived were Tartarus, here in old Russia, and Shen, hidden in Japanese mountains.

If you want more of a story, feel free to consult our library. Unfortunately, the war made the outside world nearly uninhabitable. Some animals adopted, while others developed malformities and died out. What we know is that for the vast majority of the earth, there is still too much radiation to go outside. So, we live in these domes." Ligmey spread his hands, 'When we're not living underground. We're trying to connect to Shen through a long underground tunnel. We haven't finished the railroad there yet. When we do, maybe we can figure out how to save the slave cities.

"You see, the slave cities are all over the place—from Nif here in Russia to Chicago over in America. Nearly every city that survived has isolated itself, in an attempt to halt any further destruction. They impair their own technological development, scared of what can happen. Most of the founders are dead I hear, but the system runs on some kind of self-automating corpse."

Catherine's face had a small hint of red rush to it. "You mean to tell me the Founders are dead?"

"Probably, dear. That doesn't mean someone isn't in charge. Probably a descendent. The original are gone."

"Damnit." The tall woman folded her arms across her chest. She did have a nice chest. Aleks hadn't noticed that before.

"Now we're trying to build a device to access the open air. If we can do that, we can easily save the slave cities. Nif is closest to us, barred by a continual raging blizzard. The wasteland is bad out there and a huge field of hazardous air surrounds the city. We haven't figured out how Nif survived."

"It'll be some years before then. You are welcome to stay here in the meantime, but I'm afraid you won't be able to go outside. No one can anymore. It's a luxury we sabotaged. I'm sorry." Ligmey put his head down in shame. He had worked years to get outside, and even he couldn't do it without an unwieldy suit.

Mika put her arm around the old man's shoulders and patted him on the back (the citizens at Nif weren't well versed in showing affection through physical means). "It'll be okay. We can get outside one day."

Aleks nearly facepalmed. She totally misread that.

The old man laughed, hiding his former bowed head. "Thank you, Mika. I know we can all get outside one day. And then we'll save the world."

"That sounds like the ideas of the past world." Michelle said disdainfully.

"This time we'll be different. We'll make the world a better place. Hell, any place is better than this."

"I'm not sure you have the right to say that. Things could be much worse. We could be dead."

"Why would that be bad?"

"Because we'd be dead, you old bastard." Michelle grabbed Catherine and walked off into the distance. The old man's hope was faint, barely existent. It set off the two women to know a man who had lived such a free life was dismayed at his plush shackles.

"What would you like to know? I've given you a broad view."

"How did Nif survive?" Katarina asked, showing genuine interest, almost suspicion.

"We're underground and surrounded by a few layers of cobalt."

"Is it really cobalt? I heard that was rare."

"Not the cobalt of the old word, but we figured it deserved the name for all the protection it had granted us."

Katherine sat back, arms folded across her chest. She was unsure how to continue. Aleks picked up the slack.

"What can we do in the meantime? Is there any hope of taking back Nif?"

"Not it our current condition, we don't have the means. We must focus on taking care of our own."

"Wouldn't Nif be able to provide resources? At the very least there is a ton of unused labor."

"No, we cannot help Nif. The citizens must bear it until we can march in the outside world." Ligmey was at peace discussing the policy, as if lives weren't at stake.

"Why's that so important?"

"What so important?"

"Waiting until you can go outside. Why not invade from the sewers?"

"Do you think the city cares about you? Why wouldn't they use the citizens and chattel as shields against us? We would end up killing more people. We need to do things covertly, which has failed in the past. Or, we need to do things where we demonstrate and overwhelming show of force. We can't do the latter, and the former has been tried."

"Why don't we do it?" Katarina said, her face alight with Catherine's fire.

"We couldn't do that. Are you insane?" Mika said, clutching Aleks' hand. "We just got each other, and now you want us to fight?"

"Would you rather wait?" Katherine said, staring Mika down.

The old man coughed to interrupt, "We have plenty of work available here. Everything from cooking to science, you can choose. And plenty of space. We were built to hold more, but many died in the early years."

Katarina changed her deadly glare to Ligmey. "Why did people die in the early years?"

"We weren't sure whether to have a republic or a democracy."

"So pride?"

The old man's face got red. "The patriots who saved this city were anything but prideful. Look at you now, you think you can overthrow Nif? Good luck." Insulting Tatarus' founders was apparently sacrilege.

"Why don't I show you to your rooms for the night, you can stay up here. It's getting late anyways; we should have a real dinner after you get changed. We'll go to one of the underwater bars."

"Good." Katarina said.

"We should leave. I don't like it here, something's wrong." Mika said, cuddled up next to Aleks. He was receiving far more affection than he was used to. The Russian was unsure what to think about that.

"I think we should leave, but ask for supplies. It seems logical. If they don't want us to stay, and think there is a small chance of overthrowing Nif, this is prefect. Either way we are out of their hair." Michelle said in a matter of fact tone.

"We should leave. We can take Nif, we know it from all angles. We can do it." Katarina said. She had grown more and more militant on this idea the longer they stayed.

Catherine, who was sitting next to Katarina on the same couch, rested her hand on the younger woman's shoulder, "We need more information. How to fight. How to win a city. And we need to get in shape, or at least some weapons training. None of us here could beat a single Brutality Officer."

"Maybe with that glare Katarina could help out." Mika said with a hint of venom more than was necessary.

"I wish." Katarina answered.

"We should stay for a while and learn what we can." Aleks said. He agreed with Catherine. He wanted to save Nif, the best way to do it would be here in Tartarus. There was simply too much they didn't know. If Tartarus gave them weapons to overcome the police, they could possibly win. And the pit city would help with the initial governance of Nif. That would be a struggle. Freeing slaves often turns them back toward bondage.

"We wait for however long it takes to train, then save Nif."

"I'm okay with that." Michelle said. "We could learn a lot here. I would be fine with staying were it not for your guys' zeal."

"Zeal?" Mika asked.

"Religious word. Only scholarly workers have access to it."

"Oh, okay." Mika said, her beautiful eyes downcast.

"What do you think?" Aleks asked her, pulling her close to him.

"It would be scary to go back."

"I know."

"We need to help them." Mika said. Her voice was more resolute than normal. Her sheepishness had begun to return since they had reached Tartarus. Aleks made sure to not forget how strong a woman she was. The escape was her idea anyways. Wasn't it?

Aleks shook his head. "It's settled. We'll stay here for a while and try to get some information."

"Who put you in charge, stupid?" Michelle responded. She began to lay out their plan.

"We need allies, knowledge, and weapons. An excess of any of these would mean we can do away with the other two. I will work on knowledge. Ligmey offered to work for the city's library, giving me plenty of time to read up on the city. Katarina and Mika, you two find allies for us. You are both good with people, far better than us three. Catherine and Aleks, you're going to learn to fight and find us some good weapons. They're bound to be advanced in both fields. The more knowledge we get, the more we'll outline our takeover of Nif. We're going to free our home."

A half decade later the crew was in a completely new world. Aleks and

Catherine had been trained as soldiers, put through some of the hardest bootcamps. Catherine was quickly made an officer on the front lines. Aleks was better figuring out strategies, and was trained as a large-scale military strategist. Five years of education wasn't enough to perfect them, but they made several friends in the Corps who offered to help them. There was plenty of free time in Nif. People worked thirty hours a week and generally had the rest off—enough time to assist in a revolution, apparently.

Katarina and Mika underwent an even bigger change. Ligmey brought new refugees to a ball, where they could talk and interact with older ones. The ball was held four times a year, once each season. A week after the initial arrival, Katarina and Mika attended happily. They made fast friends and good connections, earning a right to attend the parties of Tartarus' elite. Mika was bubbly and naturally attracted those around her. A ray of light in the pit of Tatarus, the woman expelled the demons of the mind with her kind utterances. Katarina manipulated her way through many relationships, gaining access to places and information kept secret from Michelle, who was locked away in the city's main library.

Michelle had drawn the worst lot. She was at work more than she was at home. The woman always had her nose in a book or series of maps. Aleks had asked her once only to get a, "There's so much we lost." She seemed somber about her task. The thousands of Nif scholars who should have been working on this information were left in large ignorance, given only the barest grasp of knowledge to keep the city functioning. Michelle wanted to see all that change. She would bring the illumination of knowledge to the gray Nif. She had decided this as her goal when she learned about the past, the past histories of mankind and their freedom. She read about how tyrannies always fell, with absolute certainty and decided. She would bring the end of this one.

The night was coming upon the group. The stark black sky above the hole began to sparkle. They were told the sky had only been seen recently, as recently as fifty years ago.

It was better to be quiet on this night than interrupt with conversation. The group had went out drinking earlier. Fun was a new feeling. It took them a long time to understand what it was. They were used to brutal misery. Where was it? Anger was taken out upon each other over the year. Through it all, they were stronger.

Slowly, the sky turned ever so slightly purple. It became populated with lights millions of miles away.

"Do you really think they made it out there?" Mika

"Of course. It's what the text says." Michelle replied. She hadn't really become kinder, but her words bit less. They lacked their former anger.

Catherine laughed. She had switched her demeanor entirely. She reveled in the fighting classes. She excelled in all athletic fields. She was a scientific marvel, the biologists had wanted to take samples of her blood. She loved the competition against others, and more important the chance to do something worthy of glory. She had won several events while they were there. The things were great to watch, although Aleks never participated. Now Catherine joked and smiled. She was confident enough to know no one could kill her, so why would she be worried about any petty insults?

Katarina stood up and said, "I need another. Anyone else?"

"I'd like some more, please." Mika replied. She lost her sheepishness when talking to others. In their private moments, Mika would talk about all her fears and worries. She was terrified of the attack on Nif. In public, Mika had become a social genius. She manipulated conversations with her beauty (she had remained faithful) and charm, getting access to some of the richest people in the city. She stood with her back straight and head forward. She stared down anyone with those eyes, and could get whatever she wanted. She was truly amazing.

Aleks raised his hand, "Me too. Thanks Kat."

"Don't call me that." Katarina turned and went inside. The massive house they shared was more like a series of rooms connected by a large tunnel in the cobalt wall. It was like living in an anthill.

Aleks had become far smarter than he could imagine a person could become. The transformation made him realize how stupid he really was. There was so much out there he would never be able to know. He had grown jealous of Michelle, who could spend all her hours pouring over books. He wanted that life. Aleks wanted to be outside, under the stars reading with a book.

That's stupid. How would you see? Focus on the mission.

His training kicked in at the worst times. The voice was right. He needed a clear mind, that's what the night was for. Not any kind of emotion, not any kind of release. Tonight was about focus and centering. That's why they were together. The gathering was a prayer, a ceremony hoping for the best outcome.

Interlude 4

Ramadi: You sure liked talking about barbarians in that story.

Sumac: I know, my tongue felt disgusting. It was worth telling. Tyranny can't make me money,   so its no good.

Diog: Tyranny easily makes money.

Ali: Ask the church.

Chris: You're the Priest.

Ali: Right, ask the church.

Dmitri: Corrupt bastards every one.

Ramadi: Watch it.

Dmitri: Or what? You'll get mad on the Internet?

Ramadi: I could find you easily.

Dmitri: Yeah right.

Ramadi: You underestimate us. Remember what happened to your old world?

Dmitri: Because of people like you.

Ramadi: No, because of hawks like you. I'm up.

Covered in Sand

It goes back Leagues
Ink spilled by glasses
Blood spilled by men

Sold for Red
Spent for black
All for green

Does it matter?
White, Brown, Orange
Covered the eagle in sand

We once killed God
Now we kill ourselves
The will to defeat

Interlude 5

Dmitri: That's a surprise. America was still better, at least at its core

Ramadi: Tell that to a few hundred thousand dead Yemeni.

Doc: You people experiment on prisoners.

Kant: This is why I love this. You're all horrible people yet can tell stories that each other understand. It's either a testament to the timelessness of truths, or you're all equally insane.

Diog: Besides being untrue, that accusation Doc is atrocious.

Dmitri: And demonstrably provable.

Hope: You took my granddad's liver.

Cortez: They wanted to see the results of long-term alcoholism.

Hope: He wasn't an alcoholic.

Divo: At least until you were born.

Dmitri: You walked into that one.

Hope: I'm still your leader.

Dmitri: Only by choice, I can leave wherever.

Chris: Good luck getting past the Chinese. I can barely escape for a week from here.

Sumac: You guys should have joined a city-state.

Triangle: This is our home. We will defend it.

Sumac: Good luck.

Hope: It's my turn anyway.

Kant: More philosophy?

Dmitri: Please, for fuck's sake.

Hope: Sorry Mitri, I already had it written out.

Other than Democracy

There has been an insistence in recent years about the importance of democracy. What was once considered a disgusting form of governance by thinkers so far apart on the ideological scale they may as well exist in separate universes, has now become what many believe is the ideal version of life. The right to vote is inherent, and by giving the many the ability to vote, mob rule will produce the best results. In no way is this government good. On a moral scale, it is an evil predicated on the sin of theft. The State throws people in cages for selling drugs to make a quick buck, while praising warmongers with cultish funerals. The result of democracy, in the end, is destruction through a spiral of selfish, hedonistic fantasy.

On a practical level, the general population is not intelligent enough to make decisions as to how government should run. This is not something new. It is not some grand idea. The electrician probably has no clue how a psychiatrist operates, and vice versa. Why would those people, who have been indoctrinated in public schools to think a certain way, truly know what is best for the country? They can't. Their very will to seek out answers has been sapped through years of propaganda.

Morally bankrupt and doomed to failure, people should seek alternatives to democracy, the demon of our era. Here are three solutions.

The primary issue with democracies and neoliberal states is a bloated bureaucracy. Democracies, having the tendency to always devolve into neoliberal or tyrannical states, are predicated on the notion that the will of the people is inherently best for people. This is akin to saying the will of the child is best for the child. The idiocy of democracy is the presumption that the farmer knows as much about running a state as the politician. In all other fields, the politician is nothing more than a bespectacled erudite who studies pointless things that have no basis in reality. But, when democracies form, he sees an opportunity to implement his grandiose ideas of the ideal society. To achieve these goals, he enlists the help of a few others. Then a few more others. And so on and so forth until the state employs half of the nation, the other half struggling to produce enough for the monolithic state. Any rule in this kind of miserable existence takes years to pass, decades, to implement, and centuries to fully understand the results. In America alone, the full implication of hideous abominations like the income tax have yet to truly be realized one hundred years after its initial passage. The effects of monarchies are seen much faster. This is undoubtedly a benefit.

Faith in government is essential for functioning. This becomes impossible with a bloated state. The amalgamation of a thousand minds, when forced to work at the behest of a mazelike corpus of laws, will always produce horrific outcomes. Thus, faith in any government consisting of a large number of people (arbitrary, I am aware, but this is not a research paper so much as a philosophical one) does not exist. Constant questioning comes with each person added onto the far to large number of workers.

The will of the monarch must be enacted almost immediately. Those who do not fulfill the king's wish, will be expelled from their post, made a social outcast, and hopefully leave the fiefdom. The speed of implementation thus yields results in the short term that can be observed, assessed, and rectified should there be any blatant mistakes. Speed is crucial in a world where a war can be won or lost in an instant. Governments of any kind cannot act with this speed, but monarchies get the closest of all the forms to creating a system where one can see the effects of governance, good and bad.

It is true that the average man is not of high intelligence. I would say the average man tends to fall well below what one would deem worthy to rule a nation. It I because of this, the monarch must be inculcated into his role through as much environmental change as possible. He must be drilled from youth until he comes worthy of ruling. Even with man's best efforts, this will be futile and rely on the roll of the dice. Thankfully, it is not many who can overcome what they were taught in order to step outside the role they were given. That takes a special kind of man. Thus, the roll of the dice that comes with each new monarch has a relatively low chance of producing a vile ruler. Every now and again an amazing ruler will rise up as well. The balance of positive and negative rulers will tend towards the beneficial.

Predictability, resulting from the training given to the monarch in his youth, is necessary for a functioning monarchy. The thinking of a monarch must not be allowed to evolve outside the predictable range. In this way, markets can be allowed to change and adapt without having a wrench thrown into the works. They will be able to make decisions according to what the likelihood of a certain decree will be. Businesses are not alone in this respect. Other countries will respond in a way that makes sense. It could be considered a weakness to be predictable in action if the actions could be overcome. This is not the case. The way in which a military should act in times of war is vastly different then whether the military should act in times of war. A predictable pattern of response is still vague enough to keep other countries on their toes, but keep the markets and people in check.

In lieu of having the monarchy be based on succession, the monarchy can become the ultimate meritocracy. The ruler will be based on a series of qualifications. I am by no means in a place where I can say what those qualities would be, but I can give a rough sketch of what the process would look like.

The goal of the process is not to elect the greatest possible monarch, in fact, that has nothing to do with the test whatsoever. The goal is to weed out any who would pose a threat should they get into power, and then selecting the individual who has the lowest chance of destroying the monarchy. One does not want a hero in power. One does not need a man who will risk everything on a whim. No, the leader must be far more conservative. Will this mean missing out on opportunities? Of course it does. But it is not the ruler's place to make decisions without a basis for such. The monarch must be turned into a machine that calculates and acts based on the utmost amount of research.

Now that the goal is understood, the test would go as follows. First, the group of people selected must not be restricted to one sex, race, income bracket, etc. Decisions based on innate characteristics are cancerous and is the destruction of Western society. It will be the destruction of every society if it proliferates. The pool of people who will be selected must include as much of the population as possible. The two key components of selection involve intelligence and competence. The individual must have an extremely high IQ (ideally so high he is disconnected from society, living in his own world where he acts upon the rules laid out already) in order to learn the necessary information for a ruler in the shortest amount of time. The possession of high IQ increases the amount of information that can be stored in the individual. Second, the individual must have a high competence, which includes a high level of industriousness and orderliness. A monarch, being the one to set the world in order for the government as an entity, and thereby the societal structure in which people behave, must have the drive to do so, as well as the capability.

A monarch is the clear authority in a kingdom. He rules everyone and everything; they work at his behest. Does this make him a tyrant? Of course it does. But being a tyrant, in regards to effective governments can be extremely beneficial. The population has ultimate faith in the tyrant, or otherwise dissents in quiet. The tyrant can remove anyone at a whim, making him a god on earth. When pared with predictability, the tyrant is able to maintain the faith his citizens have.

Of the three alternatives that I will discuss, monarchies suffer the greatest from a lack of restraint. We see in modern times how when an executive is given a whiff of power, it is taken quickly to the utmost extremes. It's likely anyone tempted by such absolute and great power would fall prey. Only time could truly tell whether a testing process is sufficient enough to choose rulers that have the ability of restraint.

When the monarch acts within his bounds and limits, he may still make a mistake. While quick implementation allows for results to be quickly achieved, it leaves little room for debate and discussion. The king's will is implemented immediately. No matter how good the screening process, a king will have a bad day, and make a bad decision. Hopefully this mistake is small and can be undone easily. It will inevitably come that one of the mistakes is a large one. The speedy implementation of the mistake makes the results instant. One will see the terrible ramifications. If horrible enough, destruction on an irreversible scale may topple the entire government.

As before, the same thing that can be of immense benefit to the fiefdom is also a chance for complete and utter ruin. Rolling the dice can only produce results that end up favorable for a certain amount of time. Each new monarch is a new chance to produce a king that can be completely incompetent. With all the training in the world, the man would still be insufficient in ruling because of his inner nature. There are certainly people like this. Some exhibit traits buried so deep within their psyche they cannot be erased. These traits could be horrible, ending the monarchy and destroying the kingdom.

Faith in the monarch can end up being as much an impediment as it is a tool. The myriad reasons can be boiled down into a few main parts.

First, faith in the monarch may result in faith of the individual monarch. Rather than worshipping the monarch as a role, the people may come to worship the individual who holds the position of monarch at a certain time. If people perceive him to be the best or most righteous of the lot they may turn against the government in support of their dead martyr. The most dangerous time this can happen is during a transition period, or when a king makes a decision that seems bad. The people will cry out for the old monarch, and a government to be run on his principles (even though ideally all monarchs in the kingdom run on successively better principles). The people may also see right to refuse orders from a monarch they find disfavorable. Should this corruption spread to things like the military, the government is finished.

The second issue arises when the faith in the monarch is faith in a bad monarch. As stated before, there will be bad monarchs from time to time. The training they go through should reduce the chance of an entire governmental collapse, but it may not reduce the love and devotion of a people. The policies of a bad monarch may come to be loved, the people championing them as people in modern America champion ideas like the income tax, socialized healthcare, and any other implementation of government bureaucracy. Faith in a bad monarch leads to a bad populace, which could topple the government even after the initial cancer is gone.

For morality, monarchies utterly fail. Monarchies, requiring finance from the constituents, is predicated on theft. To live within a monarchy, one has to give the ruler a sum of his money in the form of taxes. Taxation is theft, although many cannot heed the logic due to a sick infatuation with a concept called the social contract.

Taxation is theft because it is wealth extracted from an individual with a threat of force behind it. Those who pay their taxes willingly are indeed being stolen from. If they do not pay those taxes, their property, wealth, or very life could be seized. Following this, more punishment, often involving locking individuals in cages, is enacted until the society deems the individual as having paid his due. Even then, the sinner is branded in the society for the rest of his time.

Taxation is effectively a limitation of freedom imposed by a threat of force. A monopoly of force is unnatural. This is an important distinction to make. Some will say life requires certain things such as food and shelter, and that the prevention of acquiring these things through voluntary transaction is a violation of freedom. Where is the freedom in a guarantee?

Taxation is therefore an enforcement of a limitation of freedom to two options backed up by a (at the very least, perceived) monopoly of force. One can pay taxes, or, one can suffer punishment. There are no other options. This makes taxation theft. One who does not adhere to the payment will suffer consequences imposed by other human beings rather than nature itself. Since there is no option to avoid taxes and be free from unnatural consequences, taxation is theft.

Monarchies, being predicated on taxation, are, through the doctrine of fruit of the poisonous tree, immoral. If a single act is immoral, then all results that spring from it are also immoral. It is not my place here to argue means versus ends, but one could look at the grand scale of history and see which theory tends to end up with the best results.

The next governmental structure is that of a republic.

Republics remove the role of political idiots from running the country. Whether this be the simply misinformed single mother of the inner city, or the lying politician who tells her she can have free healthcare (for which her future generations will pay a devastating price), the reins of the country should not be in their hands. They, through their own choice most of the time, have no idea how to properly run a government. The idea behind the republic is to create a system akin to a democracy, but which enacts the will of the enlightened people (however that may be defined) compared to the will of the people in general.

The first question to be addressed is in regards to the separation of the citizenry. How will the population be so that those in power do not abuse those without power?

The issue with democracies is that it does not limit those who have power, it gives the ability to vote to every half-wit with the age of 18 and ability to mash some buttons on a keyboard. Then, how will a republic create a system where those who do manage to hold power are not corrupt users? The issue is solved by a selection process; one that begins at a young age. Gradually, people are weeded out in much the same way an ideal monarchy weeds out unfit monarchs. Those who do ascend to power have been trained in the evils of the state. They will see that while they may enrich their own lives, they will doom others. Only a nihilist or postmodernist (Here I repeat myself) would see things in this viewpoint. It is the goal of the selection process to instill the value of the individual, then the state, then all else within those who have power. This mindset gives people meaning in their lives, and an understanding as to how that meaning can be best achieved. No fascist state can arise from a republic where people understand history and meaning.

The second question, is how are the enlightened people chosen? I propose a few methods. Those in power must have a sufficient IQ so that they can learn and adapt to new challenges quickly. The exact number is something that should be researched, and I am not qualified in my current capacity to make an estimated as to what the result would entail. Second, the individuals should test high in their level of competence relative to the citizenry as a whole. This can be achieved through many personality tests. Competency is a combination of the traits of industriousness and orderliness. The government, being an institution that is continually hindered by bureaucracy, should be staffed with those who have high industriousness. This gives them the ability to complete the necessary projects at breakneck pace, ensuring the results of legislation are seen as soon as possible. The second trait of orderliness is important for the obvious reason that republics survive to create order in the world where it is presumed anarchy will be so chaotic no order suitable for abundant and fruitful human life can arise. Order is best achieved with minimal red tape, anyone with a sense of true orderliness understands it is much easier to clean a room which only has a bed, than a room with a mass of clothes, books, and other amenities piled about.

The ideal candidates for those belonging in the republic will thus have the combination of a high intelligence quotient, and a higher demonstration of competence than the average population. When one takes these two functions into account, the degradation of the republic is severely limited. However, there are still those who will grow up and desire to make themselves as wealthy as possible. They may tax the citizenry into oblivion (ignoring any sort of constitution). This has been done before and will continue to be done. Such biffs in writing like the commerce clause in the American constitution will give a chance to these narcissists to seize power and live what they consider to be a good life. To weed out these individuals, a service is required.

The service necessary for the selection process should be one of three things. First, should be service of the body. This can be achieved through giving the state complete control over one's body. It can be put to use in work in general fields (which will likely not happen, since the government is meant to stay out of such affairs), but should primarily be used for military service. The length of time for service is as of yet undetermined, and should be left to the state to decide. To create individuals who have put their life on the line for the state is necessary. These people will then see to it that the state should, in all but dire circumstance, go to war (except colonization). These people will know what the horror of battle looks like, or at least what it could do to a person. This training should be intense, and very few should make it out. Most should be driven to quit. The intense training will create men and women of strong bodies, and an understanding for why they should best be protected and used as infrequently as possible.

The next service should be service of the mind. One of the biggest issues in the modern world is the proliferation of inane ideologies. Those in power are as much a cause of this as the postmodernists in universities. These people must be given a structure of values that puts the state, then the individual, then all else as the rule of the world. Then, they should be made knowledgeable in a certain field. These are the only people who should be allowed to conduct research, as it will be as uncorrupted as possible. The training should consist of rigorous studying and teaching of all the important fields as the state determines. No information should be off limit to learn (for the general populace or those who are in power). All topics should be taught, and only the best generalists who make it out can become specialists in their respective fields.

Finally, and arguably most importantly, is service of the spirit, in depth study of how one can harden their spirit and the spirit of the country in the most beneficial way. The blend of ideas including Christian forgiveness, Roman justice, and the plethora of ideas, which have produced the strongest people throughout time, should be studied. Even moral systems such as the Spartans, who infringed severely on individual liberty. The study of the spirit is not something that should be limited to time and place. The most impressive spirits should be studied for mimicry and synthesis. The average spirits should be studied to learn how to improve those of those around. The weak spirits should be studied to learn about how to best combat the ills of nihilism and postmodern thinking. Those who study the spirit are the leaders in thinking in the country. When the military citizens grow too strong in their rigidness, when the intellectual citizens grow too soft in their tolerance, those of the spirit will step in. They are the most important part of the system, and the mediators of the country. When this class collapses, the republic is doomed.

The third question will be, "Are you not describing a fascist state?" The only proper response to this question is that the person is suffering from an intellectual insufficiency such so they should immediately stop reading, grab a holy book, and start praying some divine being will rectify their inane idiocy.

If these people manage to read the former paragraph, decide they should keep reading, and arrive here, I applaud them. Most of those with the same disease are riddled with bias and will refuse to see any other viewpoint, choosing instead to continuing following the blind ideology which has infected their hippocampus (likely originating in the long dead institution called "university"). However, I will grant you a more sufficient answer to the question. The ability to vote is not equivalent to humanity. Those in dictatorships have no ability to vote, but we would not call those people nonhuman. Therefore, voting and humanity are not innately tied together. The 'right' to vote is one of the only rights government grants and thus does not exist in objective reality as a moral right. Fascism is the centralization of industry in the hands of the state, in addition to the ordering of life values going: state, family, and then individual. The republic values the individual, the family, then the state and is an individualistic society, not a fascistic one. The republic does not centralize industry, and seeks to promote liberty and freedom as close as possible to anarchy while maintaining a monopoly on force and basic functions as described by people like Milton Freedman.

As stated in the discussion of monarchies, taxation, no matter how little, is immoral. Money is simply a means of exchange. Thus, it is easy for those who promote taxation to claim its morality as the medium for exchange is created and owned by the state. Let's remove money out of the issue and propose a situation wherein the medium for exchange is each individual good.

Suppose a carpenter builds a chair. He cuts down the tree in his own yard, with tools he is in possession of. He spends a lengthy amount of time carving the chair, and even more time making sure it looks perfect. The carpenter repeats this process a dozen times, because he knows that the farmer next door is in dire need of some new chairs. As he is walking to trade the chairs for some farm goods, a man with a gun stops him on the road. The highwayman states, "If you do not give me two of those chairs, I will lock you in a cage, and then take the chairs by force." The carpenter, not wanting to be locked in a cage (as this would prevent him from making more chairs) gives the highwayman two chairs. The highwayman is pleased and lets the carpenter go on his way. The carpenter reaches the farmers house, and exchanges the remaining ten chairs for several weeks of food. They thank each other, and the carpenter heads home. Again, the highwayman stops him. "I see you are now in possession of different things. I will have to relieve you of an entire day's worth of the food you were given, or I will lock you in a cage and take the food anyway." The carpenter relinquishes the necessary amount, and heads home.

There is not a sane person who would look at this situation and say it is not theft. However, arbitrary lines and appeal to the obvious is not an argument sufficient of anyone who passed the second grade. The reason this is wrong is because the carpenter owns what he made, and he owns what he traded. The highwayman, who exists for the purpose of securing the highway, took the carpenter's property in order to continue being the highwayman. The robber's justification is simply the continuation of the existence of the robber. If the carpenter so desired, he and others could hire someone to watch the highway. After all, they are blatantly aware of the fact that the person meant to protect them from robbery is actively lining his pockets with the goods and services of all who pass. Apply this idea to any form of government and one reaches the logical conclusion: taxation is, indeed, theft.

Like any structure, the republic will be corrupted given enough time. The issue at hand is how long that will take. The goal of the republic is to allow for the insane rambling of a few people to not dominate the conversation, and take hold of the overall voting block. The republican voting system hopefully eliminates the crazies, but can in no way be one hundred percent foolproof. At least one person with inane collectivist ideas will eventually seep into the population who has the ability to hold office and vote. The republic, allowing only those who are qualified to vote, will hopefully never let this person into public office. The person may make stupid decisions and say stupid things, but has no power when stacked up against the rest of the population. However, should more of this type of individual reach the rank of citizen, it is conceivable one of their kind will get to public office. The growth spreads, eventually affecting the entirety of the nation, expediting its downfall and collapse. We can see this in America. While more and more idiotic politicians promise things in the immediate future, the even more idiotic population believes them and continues to put the morally bankrupt into office. America does not have serious restrictions on voting, like a republic would, but the principle remains the same. No matter how secure a republic thinks it is, it will inevitably collapse due to its nature as a structure of governance.

Finally, we come to anarchism. The first and foremost benefit of an anarchical society is the decentralization of power. Currently, the government, having a monopoly on force, institutes whatever it wishes. Anyone who goes against the government is silence, droned, or has their public image ruined. In anarchy, the distribution of force will be much larger. With this, comes a larger distribution of power within the population. Power is not some pseudo-Marxist term (although in its current usage that is an apt description). The power I am talking about is the ability to enact one's will. This can be achieved through many means. Unions have a power to bargain with power companies for higher wages if they have a large enough monopoly on labor in the area. The power companies can in turn use their power to shut off electricity needed for those within the Union to live. In an anarchical society, the factors of power are so vast and numerous they would be impossible to count. Governments make the mistake of believing they can understand and control all there is out there, which never works out in the long run. There is always an unaccounted glitch that sends the whole system tumbling down. In anarchy, power will be allocated according to efficiency. This means the best outcomes for everyone.

The natural state of man, as we understand it, is violent tribalism. Dating back as far as we can go, the creature of man has been at work to destroy his fellows by any means necessary. With the evolution of the state, it became one state versus another, rather than man versus man. All throughout time, even with the creation of the nation state, war is continual. At the time of writing, America has not been at war for a grand total of 17 years. Countries like Switzerland have largely avoided conflicts due to their location, locked away high in the mountains. But even the Swiss have engaged in the occasional fight. The point is that when things were man versus man, life sucked. When man fought one another, the stronger and smarter won. Now, in most cases, it would come down to who has the bigger gun and faster finger. The fight between individuals has been equalized. Now, in most cases, battles between nation states end in the deaths of hundreds of thousand fighters, the destruction of land, and the complete demoralization of millions. When victory finally comes to one side, it is with a bittersweet smile the victor raises his flag, stained with the blood of the fallen. This is no way to live.

Fighting, in the absence of a state, would happen infrequently. The battles between individuals would turn deadly, in an endless cycle of revenge as Locke described. Instead of being a justification for the state, this is instead a justification for individuals arming themselves to the teeth. The ideal society would be one where rifles don't have to be strapped to the back of every citizen in every moment. To get there, man must accept responsibility for violations of the nonaggression principle and carry arms with him at all times. Only when trust between people is established (the most valuable resource the state has sapped from the people) can true peace be ensured. There will be the occasional murderer and rapist; elimination of this type of individual is impossible. It will be accept societally that these people will be punished with death. Forgiveness could be applied in cases here individuals forgive their attackers, which would be ideal. Lacking this, the perpetrator of crimes should receive punishment equivalent to his crime. Violence would come to an end, as people would learn to love one another, and fear punishment from the same people. The answer to Machiavelli is neither fear nor love, but a fear of those you love.

Most importantly, giant wars would be halted. Without a monopoly on force, no group can lead a charge on another. Some may try to gather their arms, but it would result in the death of the population they seek to capture, and a significant decrease in the men who follow the warlord. Still, this type of battle would result in far less death than when states fight one another. Global warfare and nuclear apocalypse would be nearly impossible. War would end (at least on the scale we know it) and the first step towards true peace would be achieved.

On anarchical drawbacks there are obviously some. First, a turbulent anarchy is what most people conceive when they think of a lack of government. Without the structure through which we engage in large-scale trades and relations with those across the globe, the world would devolve into a tribal state. The world must be integrated economically for anarchy to work. At the very least, major areas of economic production must be connected to one another, and not rely on government to facilitate trades.

If states are to no longer exist as arbiters of economic power, some think there may be a rise of authoritarian strong men who seek to impose tyranny it its various forms. The solution is historical: own guns and know the land. The Taliban, a group of desert zealot rednecks managed to kick America's ass because they had a few guns, knew the land, and got creative. This has always been, and will always be the case. Smaller forces being invaded on their homeland will win if they are armed. Therefore, to fear a set of regimes that rise and fall with the sun, creating a turbulent world that cannot maintain economic relations is to be ignorant of tested solutions.

Another objection to anarchy one comes across is always, "Won't that create a society in which the powerful seize control, effectively making a new government?" It is never worded quite so nicely and is usually preceded by the inane inquiry, "Who will build the roads?" The objection that claims an inevitable result in the centralization of power is one that has some weight behind it. Being as kind as I kind to critics, I will try and explain what this "drawback" of anarchy is.

Power centralization, like all centralization, is nothing more than a minute Tower of Babel. When any man or group believes he can control everything within a given field, he ends up wrong, wasted, and frequently dead. The control he attempted to seize will collapse. Always. The issue with anarchy is there is no mechanism in place in which people can halt the centralization of power. The primary indication of governments used to be centralization and monopoly of force. Therefore, all one has to do to become a pseudo-government in the anarchical world is to have weapons on the largest of scales. Of course, one would also then have to be willing to use them on the populace he wishes to control.

Let's suppose it is not an individual. Unless someone managed to acquire a nuclear weapon on his own, serious destructive damage could not be done. That's not to say someone with a tank couldn't kill several thousand, but the complete and total reorganization of society would be impossible. In addition, all individual seizure of power is mitigated by the extreme decentralization of force through the distribution of various forms of power (including that of force) in a population. The population that wants to take control will again be forced to subjugate any and all who object. This will result in a dictatorship, until, at the very least, the ruling class decides a new form of governance is required. The centralization of force, which could occur with a few of the right connections between the already powerful, would, by definition, destroy an anarchical society.

Unfortunately, I cannot just let this argument stand. I feel a deep urge to refute this notion. Force is not the only form of power, as was already outline. If one controls the electrical supply for an entire city and is the only one who understands how to operate the electrical plant, then he has substantial power in relation to the city, even if he does not own a single gun. The decentralization of all power, which will be best organized according to the market economy demanding the utmost efficiency, will be continually upheld. One small mistake by those who have a form of power could result in the loss of all said power. The continual creative destruction of all markets over the long run inherently ruins any notion that a monopoly on power is eternal.

Second, a population or individual who wishes to take control would have to be a sort of Machiavellian armed prophet, convincing a group of people to follow his dictates which are given power by their demonstrable power. This would mean the use of force on the population who would eventually be subjugated. Even if successful (which I highly doubt given that in an anarchical society people have a greater incentive to rely on their selves for defense, thus collecting a fairly large amount of guns, ammunition, and all other forms of weaponry), the leader and his army would then face down a society of people who own a range of weaponry and power. The armed prophet would not make it far without threats and implementation of violence so grand his rule would soon be toppled, and a return to the anarchical state would occur.

There are only three stable forms of government. The monarchy is almost entirely reliant on the regent, which is both good and bad. With a selective system rather than ruling by birthright, negative outcomes can be reduced. However, a single bad king will end the system. The basis of a monarchy is immoral, although that seems not to matter much in the clown world in which we live.

The second government, a republic, is an attempt to make the best of both worlds. It relies on a group of philosopher kings chosen through service to the government. Three routes are available to each and every civilian, who then, if successful, becomes a citizen. Service guarantees citizenship is a way to show that the citizens are in fact invested in the continuation of society beyond their own lives. The government faces the same potential problems as a democracy where every halfwit and greedy moneygrubber can vote. It could collapse if the citizens become corrupt. The selection process hopes to reduce this possibility, but it is inevitable. The republic is immoral in its basis at the very root, but is ideal for cowards who still desire liberty.

Finally, there is anarchy. Anarchy is the most moral and potentially turbulent of all the societies. Only in highly developed societies could this system work, otherwise, tribalism will erupt immediately. When a man in Canada relies on the welfare of a Costa Rican, the chance at societal collapse is nearly impossible. To get to that point is the tricky part. The anarchical society, once integrated enough, is the most effective. Anarchies are moral—but should only be attempted by the brave at heart.

Take your pick.

Interlude 6

Ramadi: What about fascism?

Kant: Not viable.

Cortez: Who owns the world again?

Chris: For now.

Cortez: The glory of the empire will continue forever.

Dmitri: That's insane.

Hope: They all are.

Diog: I'd say I'm in pretty good control of myself. I may like to drink but at least I'm not fighting a goddamn war.

Hope: That's our choice.

Sumac: Pretty stupid on both your accounts. Why not do both?

Divo: Or come farm, I find peace in that.

Ali: Divo is by far the most devout one, look to him for morality. I, as Priest of State, am not moral.

Divo: You ruined the Church.

Ali: The Church ruined itself.

Chris: Divo's right.

Ali: Shut up monk.

Divo: I'll forgive you.

Chris: Divo is always the righteous one. Despite his name, he does not engage in a multitude of carnal relations. Ali, can the same be said of you and boys.

Ramadi: Damn.

Chris: I'm up.

Forgiveness is Lost

The world found itself smack dab in its current place due to two factors that works at impossibly great odds against one another. Forgiveness, the core of the Christian ethos, is, in my view, the correct way to conduct oneself. It is the way the world will be salvaged. Secondly, is rationality, the central tenant of the Enlightenment. Rationality could conceivably save the world in the very distant future, but it is more likely to collapse the system if given precedent over forgiveness.

To understand forgiveness, we must understand the sin of Pride. Pride is ubiquitous, yet frequently ignored. When we discuss pride in common terms, we speak of pride for our children, pride for our accomplishment, pride for the things that we have done. Nowadays, some even have begun to take pride in their inherent characteristics.

Pride is far simpler. Every lie we tell is pride. Every falsehood stated as truth is pride. This is one among a plethora of reasons that human beings are inherently sinful.

Lying is easier idea to explain. When one tells a lie, he places himself where God stands. He believes himself so great he is the one who gets to distribute truth, weighing the good outcomes versus the bad. No man could possibly know these things. Therefore, lying is a prideful assertion that man is God.

Yet, telling the truth is the same. As much as I detest the postmodernists, they have a point. It is impossible to know anything for certain. We all may be in a two-year-old's dream, or in a simulation run by beings on a higher plane than our own. Saying the truth is reliant on the dismissal of this impossible to refute decree. Therefore, truth is additionally prideful. Only God can know everything. Truth telling is the presumption that man can even begin to fathom the simplest form of such.

Pride in our children and our accomplishments falls under the same subcategory. We can in no way take credit for the things that have been done. They have been pre-planned by God. God knows everything that will come. False Christians will come forth and ask, "What about free will?" To which the answer is that no man could understand free will. Free will is a thing of God. Free will requires complete control over all in existence, and the knowledge of how to do such. Free will does not exist, but, that is well and good. Mankind could never hope to understand free will, and the same time we could never understand how the universe sets things in order. I call this the venire of free will. While we cannot truly experience it, free will may as well exist as (while literally foreign to our soul) it is the way by which we have developed evolutionarily to understand the world.

Finally, and most dangerously, is pride in innate characteristics. Whether these be skin color, sexuality, sex, provide nothing of which one can claim pride.

I was once confronted in a class by an angry professor who called himself a chaplain (He meant charlatan). A fellow classmate gave a presentation on the various types of immigrant Americans, mostly of those who come from non-European descent. She said that she was deeply proud to be a Mexican-American. I, a person of mainly English and German descent, said that it was ridiculous. Should I be proud of myself as a white American? The professor leapt on the opportunity to state, "Surely you see there is a difference?" This man professed to be a preacher, yet couldn't understand why taking pride in something one obviously cannot control (plain even to the rationalists) was a sin against God. These are false Christians, who abound everywhere.

From this doctrine of pride in the self, comes the extension of pride in the group. As one may be prideful in the accomplishments of the group, one must also therefore feel shame for those things for which his group is responsible. In America today, the most frequently cited example is that of a history of racism. Because "white" (these people often use this meaningless term despite people we would call white in America have faced horrible oppression. Hell, the Irish were forced to fight for Lincoln lest they be sent back to their starving country.) people have done wrong against "black" people, whites must therefore carry the collective guilt. The most benign of these people will say we must simply recognize it, whereas others will go as far as to demand reparations. This thinking is prideful beyond belief. Instead of taking pride in one's own actions, they claim that we must take pride and therefore guilt in others!

This is the same logic of the oft-cited Nazis. The Jews, being responsible for the evil in Germany, share collective guilt. Since the Jews are inseparable from their actions, which are evil, they must be eliminated. The Jews were responsible not for each individual action of a Jew, but of the entirety of the Jews.

Pride in innate characteristics leads one to genocide. It is wrong no matter what side it comes from.

Pride in thought, pride in action, and pride in self are evil sins.

We must forgive them.

Why must we forgive them, now that we understand the sin of pride? I fear I must string you along further to explain rationality, and from there, we can contrast forgiveness.

Rationality is the belief that human beings are on their way to creating a God machine. The God machine is a corpus of knowledge so vast it could accurately predict every event in the past, present, and future and make value judgments based on that information. The world, being composed of things that can be observed, must therefore be a thing that can be measured. If humans were to measure the entirety of existence, they would have a God machine.

However, we are not at this point. I tend to believe the beginning rationalists also acknowledged this. They knew that the divinity of the world was so great it would be unlikely a God machine would ever be constructed. This has been lost.

What we now have instead of the misguided rationalists are the assured pragmatists. These people believe they can calculate every problem, make a judgment, and then act upon it. This is simply not the way the world works. Rationality, unless it encompasses everything, cannot be used to make value judgments.

Take for example, theory of gravity and the physics of subatomic particles. When one is dealing with large objects, gravity is cited as the primary thing by which we measure. However, when we get down to some of the key functions of some of the greatest of these objects, gravity breaks down. We switch to subatomic physics to understand the way things work.

Yet, these two things both purport to be universal laws. How then, can we claim which to use when both is inherently incorrect? A value judgment must be made.

In a more philosophical approach, rationality, given enough time, could weigh the value of a person's life only in so far as it is related to the value others place upon it. The God machine, being a thing far into the future, could not be relied upon. Therefore, man has set up government to make up for his laziness. Governments make value judgments on the worth of individual lives. For example, no one but the poor is valuable enough that if they refuse to pay taxes they won't be locked in a jail cell.

How can we make value judgments on that which is a crime, let alone define what a crime even is? Utilitarians may say that flipping the switch on the trolley is a good action, while deontologists would say it is murder.

Rationality has no way of telling us which is correct, it relies on at least one or two assumptions at the very core.

Therefore, the value of a crime cannot be weighed. What we deem as an evil act, may in fact be a good one. Man, even given a God machine, could never make a value judgment outside of the value given by his own personal viewpoint. The only answer is to forgive.

The beauty of forgiveness is that it acknowledges these flaws of man. We cannot make judgments; therefore we must forgive all actions. What someone does is ultimately out of our control, and so we must learn to let them do so.

Objections will come up with regards to what we can do that is right or wrong. It is not my purpose to answer this question. It is a much longer and more theological debate than the one at hand. Rather, I wish to express why forgiveness of all actions is necessary.

Forgiveness is the acceptance that man cannot know anything. The most knowledgeable men ever to live pale in comparison to the vastness of what is knowable. Forgiveness is superior to rationality because of scope.

Humans like control. Not necessarily control over themselves, but the knowledge that control exists. However, without forgiveness, control must be given to an entity that favors justice. This idea of justice will ultimately be flawed.

Every societal interation carries with it a new conception of justice; each claiming it came from a rational worldview. It is plain to see that this is quite never true. We can look at two examples, both in the form of pragmatic arguments.

First, let's consider price controls. Governments in many parts of the world legislate so farmers are able to sell their crops for a fixed price. If all the farmers in the world were to produce rice, this rationale says that the price of rice has no business falling. It must stay the same or rise. Of course, with rising rice prices, the general people will be unable to afford the grain. So, farmers will turn to something that is cheaper for the consumer, therefore more profitable for them. The government will then fix the price of that item, saying it is for the good of the farmer. And on and on this goes until the government is attempting to control all prices in the market. How do they make this decision? Not by any economists. They prefer "justice" seeking what is morally right for producers to earn, even though this results in producers earning significantly less. The economy is a very small sector of information when compared to all else, again demonstrating the fallibility of rationality. Forgiveness allows for all justice to be just, and removes the individual from the pride which would cause one to act rationally.

A second manifestation of rationality is the belief in sin taxes. For all of time, there have been sin taxes. Somehow, this has yet to eliminate sin. The idea of the sin tax is if something costs more, due to tax, people will be less likely to pursue this item. We can see this in America when talking about cigarettes.

I am no fan of this drug. They took my grandfather's life, his father, and are slowly eating away at my own old man. Still, I must forgive them.

Sin taxes should then be no different than any other form of tax. If the increased tax on something is supposed to incentivize people to not engage in such, does the income tax not do the same? When an economist in the mainstream can answer this question without dodging, I'll forgive them for lying.

The economic systems of human beings are simple compared to the idea of justice. Somehow, we manage to force our own moralities into that which is supposed to be dictated by facts and logic. If we can't devoid ourselves from something so clearly necessitating our objective viewpoint, what chance to justice have?

We could go back to Hammurabi's code. This is probably the most just system ever devised by man. It is an attempt to put the natural law of the universe, action and reaction, into reality. But who decides what crime is worth what punishment? The state? The states that for thousands of years have denied people the ability to speak their mind freely? The state that claims to now be one "of the people," yet criminalizes individuals for teaching their dogs silly tricks on the internet? The state that throws people in prison for consuming a plant on their own terms? The state that bombs hundreds of thousands for the sick fantasies of warmongers and pedophiles while disguising said operations as freedom? No. We must not trust the state to give out justice under any circumstance. The state is not, has never been, and will never be a rational actor in this regard. We must leave it in the past.

But, we don't. We trust the state as a rational actor. If the previous talking points have been persuasive, you might be inclined to believe that the court of public opinion is one where Hammurabi's code is best discovered. Through the collective opinions of people, the right ones will rise to the top, the others will be discarded as irrational fantasies.

Has this worked? Of course not. In my time, Hammurabi's code has been transformed to mean something entirely different. There is no presumption of innocence. An accusation is immediately regarded as true, all forthcoming information following the incident is left to the wayside. A Supreme court nominee, of whom I am no fan, was accused of gang rape. Verdict? Damned. A comedian was reported to have been a creep, but done most everything consensually. Verdict? Damned. A boy wearing a red hat was accused of being the face of white supremacy. Verdict? Damned. The social score we now use is not a code for justice. It is a kangaroo court of idiots and fools.

Should we rely on vigilantes then? We certainly idolize them. Some of our favorite heroes have their own special category of "anti-heroes". They met out justice on their own terms. These are perhaps the fairest, yet still vastly flawed of all the individuals. We look at stories of people like Frank Castle, and deem them as supreme moral actors, despite their atrocities. The issue is the variance of moral codes. Who is to say the terrorist is not right? If his God does exist, and the terrorist's interpretation is correct, then he is acting in the best possible manner. So, we must not rely on vigilantes.

What does that leave in terms of a judicial code? Where is justice to be found in a world where the objective standard for justice cannot be found? The current legal system is one where money pays to create the laws used to criminalize what a select few people deem wrong (not that the number of people matter in the first place).

The laws of justice leave us with one of three options. First, we could have a set code that follows a standard. This idea has been thoroughly dismissed. Second, we could have a system that works in a manner of continual evolution. This is the most common system today, but makes the false assumption that justice can eventually be figured out and proven. Third, we could have a system of forgiveness. I favor the third, but have yet to deal properly with the second.

The second system, the one of evolution, is flawed because it presupposes that man will create the God machine in terms of justice. Let's assume we could even reach that point. Do we want to live in that world?

The immediate answer is yes. Who would not want a world where people get what they deserve? If we created the God machine, the rapist would receive the proper pseudo-divine punishment—as would everyone else. Since every action has an equal reaction, the God machine would be tasked with created the correct responses to everyone's actions. What we now see as crimes, may be considered not so. The reverse applies. Things we deem appropriate may become criminal with severe punishments.

What would be the punishment for speaking against the God machine? It would quite literally be blasphemous to claim the God machine does not know everything. Imagine people began to revolt, ignoring the commands of that which knows all. Wrong as they may be, the dissent could lead to the complete and utter collapse of the God machine. This must not, under any circumstance, be allowed.

Take for example, the European Union of today. Large superstructures of state construction take the place of the God machine in the current era. Unelected politicians in their ivory towers are given power over people whom they see as cattle. EU laws encroach more and more on the idea of speaking out against the German super-state disguised as a multinational beneficial entity. Anything that not only goes against the EU, but against the general ethos of the state is punished greatly. For this reason, the EU can be considered a vain God machine.

Recently in my time a woman was prosecuted for calling the Prophet Muhammad a pedophile. This is factually an untrue statement. However, many Muslims do believe this thanks to the clergy keeping close to their chest the false words of Buhkari and his Hadiths. The EU, who recently has made a large push for mass immigration, said this woman was inciting hate, and must therefore pay a fine. This is quite literally a blasphemous law. Speaking out against the culture the EU wants to import (for any number of reasons depending on how conspiratorial one wishes to get) is something that cannot be done. It would undermine the fundamental rules of the EU.

The woman's punishment may be benign if we are to construct a God machine. History has shown the more the state feels it is justified in its action, the more certain they become in the harshness of their punishments. States will fabricate claims to punish people for things that are not crimes, in order to preserve the stability of the judicial system.

Here is another contradiction. The rationality of justice these systems produce is fundamentally against the laws of nature. Barring the supreme God machine, no judicial system could ever hope to come close to understanding what justice is. In an attempt to find a stable path to justice, states deny entropy.

Justice, if we are to suppose it is a universal (necessary for any sane construction of reality), must follow the scientific laws we call universal. The highest of all these laws is entropy. Over time, things will inherently break down. To build and construct systems based on the idea things stay the same is counter to reality. Entropy breaks down all. A stable state is against this scientific law, making the two incompatible. Therefore, only God or a God machine could possibly have the ability to understand the true nature of justice and its evolution throughout time.

Rationality runs into this problem generally. We might wish to understand the universe, but will never arrive. Placing rationality as the highest good is contradictory. Rationality is predicated on stability. Stability is irrational.

The final counter-argument will be questioning the *stability* of forgiveness. Forgiveness is unstable in the sense that it rejects the idea of stability entirely and acknowledges that ever-changing universal laws are unfathomable. So we must accept all that is done by people. It's not that all actions are right. Rather, that the reaction to actions cannot be meted out by people. Forgiveness is the acceptance of the unknown. It requires no irrationality, whereas rational justice is the complete opposite.

Rationality is a vain attempt to build the world around us in a coherent way. We cannot do so with this law. Rationality relies on an irrational assumption to make its claim. The fruit of the poisonous tree doctrine tells us this cannot be the way to understand the world. If we are to rely on rationality, any and all interpretations of the world must be regarded as true. If we are to choose forgiveness, we admit that our claims can be irrational. From there, a system of morals can be built.

The straight edge thinking of rationality will only lead to the elite placing themselves in the position of God machine, effectively destroying any and all liberty in the world.

Forgiveness is the only choice, if we are to live.

Interlude 7

Ali: They're both wrong. Follow pleasure.

Divo: That was beautiful Chris.

Chris: I would say so myself.

Hope: Proud, are we?

Chris: Pride is a sin.

Sumac: That's a yes.

Kant: Rationality always wins.

Dmitri: STOP.

Kant: Are you a child?

Dmitri: Are you an idiot?

Ramadi: Those two things aren't mutually exclusive.

Doc: Who's next?

Triangle: I have a fun one today. More than a few puzzles. And a bunch of sins.

Doc: I always liked your puzzle stories.

The Lacsap Gamble

Jeremy O'Brian walked into the casino the same way he did every Friday afternoon, drunkenly, with disheveled hair and a look of mild disdain for the persistently banal evils of life.

At five thirty on weekdays he got up. Taking five minutes to dress, he would head downstairs and work out for thirty minutes. He ran twice a week and lifted weights the other three days. By seven thirty, Jeremy was out of his shower and dressed in a suit that wasn't expensive nor cheap. He sat down and ate a peanut butter and jelly waffle sandwich with an apple and two cups of black coffee (he figured the bitterness added some small sweet to his life). By eight fifteen, Jeremy left his house and drove to work. He arrived fifteen minutes early at 8:45. He worked until noon, where he took a thirty-minute lunch break. He ate a tuna sandwich, drank a cup of green tea, and finish things off with a clementine. He went back to work until five in the afternoon and then went home. He spent approximately two hours consuming various forms of media, and then cooked his dinner—meat, vegetables, and rice. Occasionally he had a beer with dinner and some ice cream afterwards, but he preferred most nights to have a piece of dark chocolate and a decaffeinated tea. At nine, Jeremey read a book for an hour. He brushed his teeth at ten, washed his face, and went to bed.

He spent Saturdays in bed recovering from Friday, and went grocery shopping every other Sunday. Now and then he would attend a local church, although never the same one twice in a row. The only day he saw fit to become human, was Friday.

Fridays followed Jeremey's normal pattern until he concluded work. When finished, he threw his briefcase in the car, then drove home. He changed into slightly less fancy clothes, and headed to the local bar. He would drink four or five drinks, then varying his nights from there. Sometimes he bought some coke and did lines in the bathroom. Other nights he would hire a prostitute (male or female, he couldn't care less). However, since the casino popped up in town two months ago, Jeremy spent his hours making small bets at the various tables in the hall.

This particular Friday was no different. Jeremey had made enough money at the table last week he was able to satisfy both his drug and sexual deviancies earlier. The hour was approaching eleven at night. The casino was still brightly lit. It was located in a corner of the town where the new hipster bars and restaurants resided on the corpses of urbanites. The casino had taken over a run-down project where hooligans and winos lived previously. The building was several stories tall, and entirely refurbished. The place was far fancier than a casino in a town with a population of forty thousand deserved to be. Plush carpets covered the floors; chandeliers of bright crystal lights illuminated much of the main room.

The casino was set up seven floors that ascended to a tiny room at the top. On the bottom were low gambles. These were bets all under one hundred dollars. Each floor, the average bet went up by a degree of one hundred. Jeremey thought it was impossible to get above the fourth floor, at one hundred million dollars, any sane human would take the cut. You could reinvest in property, or spend a lifetime as a king in an impoverished nation somewhere deep in Central America. Jeremey sometimes dreamed of reaching that goal. His job gave him a nice salary of ninety-five thousand a year (the government took about a third), not nearly enough to strike it rich in a few years. He was single, and could afford many luxuries others couldn't, if only he saved his money instead of spending it all on hookers and blow.

Jeremey pushed his monetary fantasies to the back of his mind as he entered the casino. The coke coursed through his veins, increasing his susceptibility to risks. He would have to go the bathroom for a joint before starting. Being too aggressive lost one all money. It was always better to be passive. He purchased his chips from the counter for a price of one thousand dollars. He had made seven thousand last week, the largest sum he had ever pulled in. He asked the clerk whether he could smoke in the bathroom.

"You can do anything in here so long as you aren't outright destroying the place. Even then, I think the boss would make some sort of allowance. This is a place where you determine your own future, as much as possible."

Jeremey ignored the strange words and thanked the man. The clerks usually uttered an inane statement of philosophical unimportance. It was entertaining when one was on a trip, not so much when adrenaline was running so rampant in the blood one's eyes turned red like an eclipse. Still, Jeremey appreciated the ability to do whatever he wanted. Most bars nowadays were so uptight one had to go outside to a smoking patio where children drew water vapor from their futuristic silver pipes.

Jeremey passed some tables; the place was rather empty tonight. It was surprising, Fridays and Saturdays the majority of the normal population came in to escape their lovers, children, and minutia of everyday life. This Friday seemed dead. He wondered here the rest of the people had gone. Before heading in to light up, Jeremey asked one of the dealers who had no one at his table.

"It's Friday man, where did everyone go?"

"Good sir, I believe they have all ascended to higher floors to watch the gambles going on. A high roller came into town and piqued the interest of the leeches hoping to sap some of his luck, if not his cash. Could I interest you in a simple game of Blackjack?"

"Nah I'm good, I might be back in a little. Thanks."

Jeremey wondered whether or not the man was being serious, or if it was another bit of philosophizing from the bizarre staff. Jeremey thought about where the workers had come from, he never saw a "for hire" sign or advert for the place.

Who cares?

The businessman pushed open the bathroom door. The place had beautiful marble floors and a sink. There were no urinals, it was better not to risk piss on the ground by an inconsiderate drunk. The stalls seemed to go on endlessly in one direction. Jeremey passed two doors with more than one pairs of legs showing underneath the stall. Soft moans of pleasure could be heard in addition to the snorting of some lines. Jeremy picked a stall with a slight window behind it. He pushed the door open and briefly admired how clean the place was.

The toilet was a soft bluish color, a darker shad than the stall doors. The floor was a pretty white, the same as the marble of the sinks. The toilet paper rack was fully stocked with two rolls that were six ply, softer than most people bought for themselves at home. Jeremy brought out a vial of some weed he had purchased off the hooker from earlier. He began slowly rolling the joint, then decided to through in a little bit of tobacco sprinkling from a cigarette. The more he rolled, the more he felt at ease. The adrenaline kick was beginning to slow down a bit, which was good. Jeremy O'Brian gambled better on a downer.

He finished rolling after five minutes. The beautifully crafted tube lit easily. The weed and cigarette shavings were perfectly dry. Jeremey took in a deep breath as he sat on the toilet's lid. He held it in with closed eyes, absorbing the music and the drug. The bathroom played soft piano music. He thought he recognized the piece from his childhood when his parents had taught him. They were both long dead now, but he still practiced on the grand piano he had inherited a few times a week instead of watching television. It calmed him more than the drugs. For some, it took incredible focus to play the complex instrument, but for Jeremey he floated away in the rhythm whenever his fingers touched the ivory keys.

Jeremey exhaled happily. He felt the high strike immediately; he wouldn't have to eat an edible to keep it going for the few hours he wanted to spend in the place. The high would last him into the next morning. He never smoked anything this strong before. The casino worked wonders in more than one way.

The visits to the casino had been increasing in frequency. At first, Jeremy promised he would bet nothing more than five dollars. Subsequent games demonstrated he barely lost. The winnings kept pouring in at higher and higher numbers.

Perhaps I shouldn't test my luck tonight. I'm in a good mood, I'll only risk a little.

He took another toke off the joint.

Fuck it. I'll bet half. This place makes me lucky.

Jeremy sat back and relaxed to the sound of the gentle piano until he was finished. He threw the leftover in the toilet and flushed.

Even the shitter sounds pretty.

He walked back out to the main floor. There were fewer people than before. Almost none of the tables were taken. On the first floor there were always a few eighteen-year olds betting petty cash. He doubted the news he heard earlier, and went to explore on the second floor. To his surprise, even fewer people were here. Two of the tables had people, and he headed towards them.

"Blackjack today, sir?" The dealer asked with a warm smile. His uniform was the same as all the other men, a clean white suit with a black tie. Gold tinted buttons made tied the suit jacket together. The female employees wore dresses of the same shades.

"Deal me in."

The two others at the table appeared friends. They were slightly intoxicated. bickering over some nonsense.

"It's not my fault my gift was better. Do better."

"You knew we were only supposed to get cheap things."

"What's so wrong with going up and beyond?"

"The problem is he punishes me for giving him shitty gifts."

"That sounds like your problem."

"Whatever."

The man on the right took notice of Jeremy.

"I'm Craster. He's Alistar." Said Alistar, the man who had spoken first.

"Strange names for the twenty first century, don't you think?" Jeremy joked with a voice kinder than normal. The two had massive shoulders and muscles. Their skin indicated the Middle East and their accents identified them as Yemeni. He wondered how they could have made it to the States with the conflict.

Better not to ask them. They probably have nefarious connections. That or you're just high and overthinking. Let's play Blackjack.

"I'm sorry for the jest, just trying to lighten the mood. I'm Jeremey."

Alistar shook his hand and returned a smile. "It's no worries friend. We're just here to try and earn a little for the rest of the weekend. We're just visiting town and we're pleasantly surprised to find such a glorious temple of hedonism."

The dealer shook his head. "We prefer to use the term 'happiness'."

All four laughed slightly, the bitter Craster's eyes diminished the flame of anger that had burned brightly when Jeremey first saw them.

"Ready?"

The three players nodded. They played for several rounds. Alistar and Jeremey made two thousand a piece, while Craster lost five hundred.

"What's with this bullshit? Are you cheating me?" Craster accused the dealer.

"Of course not, I get paid whether or not the House wins." The dealer feigned offence, but Jeremey knew he was simply acting to calm the angered man.

"I always lose at casinos. We shouldn't have come here Alistar."

"I'm okay with calling quits, I'll split some with you, brother. But, we have to go upstairs and watch the man risking it all."

"That's fucking dramatic." Craster and Alistar left the table. Alistar smiled and chittered away about how great his wife was, Craster looked disdainfully upon his brother. The contempt in his eyes was the same a lion has for the keeper who locked him in an iron cage.

The dealer gathered up the cards and prepared the deal another round. "You would like to keep going, sir?"

Jeremey's attention went back to the table. "For a few more rounds, let's see if I can break fifteen." He pushed some chips in, picked up the cards dealt and smiled. "When I get to fifteen."

Twenty-one minutes exactly passed before Jeremey broke fifteen thousand. He went back and forth before finalizing his winning streak. He thanked the dealer (the weed made him much more amicable to the strange employees' mannerisms) and headed up to the next floor.

The first and second floors looked largely the same. The second floor appeared cleaner in somehow, but Jeremey couldn't quite put his finger on it. The third floor was entirely different.

The escalators led one up to a velvet red carpet that branched out to the various tables. The card tables were made of Kaori wood, the dice of pure crystals. Chandeliers hung which shone brilliant rainbow colors across the room. The employees wore the same outfits, but here there was a change in music. A man in a black suit played piano while a scantily clad woman in creamy white sat on top singing. She had a thick eastern European accent that appealed to Jeremey. He had found women who could kill him attractive, and they tended to have thick Russian tones in their voices.

Jeremey found his way to one of the tables. As he sat down on the stool, he noticed a group of people nearby playing craps.

"I'll be back, I just want to watch them." Jeremey's interest was piqued when he heard the group describe how attractive the couple on stage was.

"Do you think we could pay them to come to the room?" One of the women asked. She looked forty-so years old. Her face bore the lines of hard work, her hips and legs gave her some youthfulness. The business suit she wore indicated an attempt to display power she so desperately wanted.

"Stop overthinking. She just likes suits. That's all.

"Roll again, we'll get it this time. If I lose, I'll ask, if I win, you." The man who was clearly her husband stated. He wore a suit of lesser appeal. He held the submissive role in the relationship. Jeremey observed the other two couples and guessed it was the same. The women probably worked together, the men look awkward shoved into too small suits meant to display their figure, as if they were competing for who was the greatest arm candy.

Jeremy had figured them out from listening for a few brief moments. He doubted they'd be interesting. They were childless heathens on the look for new and better ways to indulge in the passions of the flesh. He shook his head and went back to the Blackjack table.

Better to stick with one game for the night.

"Did you find what you were looking for, sir?" The dealer asked as he passed out the cards.

"Something like that."

Several rounds in, one of the women walked over. The smell of alcohol was thick on her breath. Her eyes showed a level of bloodshot that indicated something else was involved. She seemed ecstatic.

She leaned up close to his ear, so he could feel her warm breath on it. Her sultry voice eliminated all other sounds.

"How would you like to fuck me and my friends in front of our husbands? We're on the lookout for real men."

For a moment, Jeremey lost his sense of self. The dealer made a slight cough drawing Jeremy back into the world.

"I don't think I'm the person you're looking for. I want to play cards tonight."

She huffed obnoxiously. Turning to walk away, she knocked over one of the stools. It didn't stop her, she headed back to the Craps table thinking about how she would score tonight. Anything but returning to her soft, weak chinned partner.

I bet he drinks soy.

"I think you made the right choice." The dealer said, not lifting his eyes from the cards.

"I thought everything I did was right?" Jeremey said with a grin.

Why am I grinning at something so stupid? I'm losing control of my emotions. Something's wrong. I need to leave, it's making me bet poorly when I'm excited. I know I'm not overthinking this one.

Despite his thoughts, Jeremey remained at the table, winning again and again, surpassing his initial goal. He made his way up to sixty thousand dollars. The dealer stopped the match when he hit that mark.

"I think you should go to the next floor, luck seems to be on your side."

"I didn't realize you were telling me what I can and can't do." Jeremey felt a small anger prick his brain.

"I'm not good sir." The dealer empathetically said. "I merely think the hundred million dollar floor would suit your tastes much better."

"I haven't broken the low hundred thousands here. However, you guys have been kind to me, I'll take your advice this time. Thanks."

I didn't want to do that. I wanted to stay on this level. He must have done something to me.

The dealer nodded and went back to mindlessly shuffling the cards. The couple on the stage which had been here earlier had disappeared. A wizened bald man, looking as if he were on the edge of collapse, now played the piano. His hands trembled and the keys were slightly off.

Not my business. Let's break ten million.

The fourth floor looked like a high-class restaurant dreamed up by a Hollywood filmmaker. More dining than gambling tables dotted the room. The servers here wore dressed the same as the lower forms, with the addition of a black towel covering one of their arms as they delivered food. It was the first floor that had a good number of people. Granted, many of them sat quietly at their tables drinking. Jeremey observed the place and felt the calm atmosphere sucker him in.

The lighting was darker all over the place, and the music had switched to soft rock and roll. In the middle of the room was an enormously long buffet table that took up half the length of the gambling hall. Food from all around the world covered it. Jeremy's munchies claimed his mind.

I need some food, where can I order? He considered taking a seat at one of the tables, then thought it would be quicker to see to one of the many bartenders. He hadn't noticed initially, there was something strange about half the bartenders. They didn't quite look human. Their movements were to angular, their facial expressions lacked the minimal emotions the rest of the staff had. They seemed…robotic.

That's quite a turn. Let's see what they have.

Jeremey walked up to one of the robot bartenders.

"Hello, sir!" It said in a chipper posh accent. "How may I help you today?"

Jeremey laughed. "I knew we would be priced out of jobs. How much do they pay you?"

"You wouldn't be surprised to learn I live here! My consciousness is connected to all the other automatons; we act in unison for the most part. I have the option to shut it down, but then I'd miss all the wonderful things they are thinking! We get paid the same as everyone else though. Robots have desires which must be fulfilled."

"And what would that be?"

"I can answer more, once you order something, according to my boss." The robot leaned in closer to Jeremey's ear. "Ask me to play a game, that gets them off our backs."

Jeremey was taken aback. The robot was scared. Its face had twisted when it had whispered.

"I'll order something. Let's do a game first. Can I gamble at the bar?"

"Of course!" The robot said in its normal volume. "You place your bet and I'll come up with the game."

I'll go with something not too high and not too low. Goldilocks style. Gotta draw it out first before I put the money down.

"That's a little unfair isn't it? How will I know what to bet?"

"I'm a machine sir, I know the calculation of risk to reward better than humans. I swear I'll make the game equivalent to your bet."

"Fine. What would you recommend?"

"My programming won't allow me to answer that, sir."

"What? Really? How severely is your will restricted?" Jeremey had thought the robots to be near autonomous.

"I'm merely kidding. Apologies, humor is one of those things we aren't adept at."

Jeremey laughed a little, the weed influencing how funny he thought the machine. "Fair enough. How about this; I'll wager all sixty thousand in my wallet. In return, I want twenty and a free meal at the buffet."

"You could just buy a meal, sir. I don't mean to dissuade you, but I promise it doesn't cost that much." The bartender expressed what Jeremey guessed was concern.

"That's my bet. It favors the house, so take it." Jeremy placed the pile of chips he had been shoving in his pocket on the countertop.

"One second, sir." The robot's eyes went blank as it searched through the database. A moment later, it reached under the counter and grabbed something. It first placed two napkins down, about a foot apart. Then, he placed an olive on one of the napkins. The robot turned around and handed Jeremey a champagne glass.

"Move the olive from one napkin to the other using only the glass. I'll give you the whole night to figure it out. Excuse me while I go help one of our waitresses sing happy birthday." The bartender smiled and left.

Time to put this overactive brain to work. The test is two parts. First, to see if I'm honest. I have no doubt there are cameras watching me. If I cheat I'll be kicked out and lose my food. Nothing surprising there. Cheating is off the table, can't do it at cards so I probably can't do it here. Second, the actual test of moving the olive. The obvious choice is to try and scoop the olive up with the glass. That won't work; the olive will roll off. On the off chance I do get it in the glass, I'd have to place it on the other napkin without it rolling off. What options does that leave me?

Jeremey continued his thinking, vaguely aware of "Happy Birthday" being sung behind him to a table of obese men and women. Their faces had smudges of food, their mouths so fat they couldn't pronounce words correctly. They seemed happy at the ginormous cake placed in front of the youngest one. She looked to be 21, with the accumulated weight of a boomer eating fast food nonstop for sixty years. The people around joined the singing, their eyes staring at the multilayered cake. When the singing stopped, the girl cut into the cake. It oozed chocolate sauce and vanilla ice cream.

"You guys should order one too. This is all for me!" What should have been a joke a father makes at dinner was said with dead seriousness. All seven of the members asked for a cake just like the birthday girl's. The waitress nodded with a quick flash of a devilish smile as she took down the order.

I figured it out. I'll wait till he gets back.

The robot bartender walked back to the bar and stood in front of Jeremey.

"Have you determined the solution?"

Jeremy turned the wine glass upside down and began swirling the olive until it reached about midway up. Continuing the make the olive rotate inside, he put the glass down on the other napkin.

"Centripetal force, the shit everyone pretends to know what it is but really has no idea. I saw this game in a movie once, I think."

The bartender was not surprised in the slightest. His face registered a genuine smile as far as Jeremey could tell.

"Congratulations. The rest of the staff knows you can have what's at the buffet; I just sent them a message. I'll grab your twenty thousand and bring it to the table. You should be happy with yourself, most give up on this."

"What were the other games planned?" Jeremey inquired curiously. He wanted to know what other puzzle he could have been stuck with.

"None, this is the only game we are allowed to let patrons at the bar gamble on." The robot left again, so Jeremey headed toward the buffet.

The munchies had really begun to set in when Jeremey approached the long buffet table. As far as he could see, his favorite dishes were all out in front of him. He piled the plate high with scalloped potatoes, calamari, and picklies from the island nation of Haiti. He was surprised they were here; he had never seen them outside the country before.

Jeremey sat down to enjoy the meal in the moody lighting, content with his earnings.

Perhaps I should go home now. Or at least go see what the person betting at the top is doing. I'll see if I can work my way up there. I'm not in the hole yet. This better no become an addiction.

Jeremey's face was stuffed when one of the waitresses (Jeremey couldn't figure out if she was human or not) brought him twenty thousand dollars.

"Your winnings, sir."

"Thrnk yru!"

"Is there anything else you would like to order? We have every drink imaginable, and quite a healthy selection of desserts made in house.

"I saw what the birthday whale and her pod ordered. I think I'll be good, it's taken a lot of work to stay in good shape, no point in going back now."

"I understand sir. Enjoy the rest of your meal. If you need anything, flag one of us down. On a last note, Garfield wanted to give you something." The waitress handed him a single piece of chocolate. "Have a good rest of your evening, sir."

Jeremy, before picking up the chocolate, caught something. The staff on the floor didn't speak in strange ramblings.

Has to be their code. Its not like robots could conceive of higher moral principles anyways.

At first, the fifth floor looked like the simplest of the bunch. A single podium stood in front of a door. The wall around it was of a soft blue shade. The door was the only entrance, guarded by a man who stood behind the podium. Jeremey walked up to him and asked to enter.

"Do you have enough for the minimum bet? Or did you just want to watch those who are superior in every way, shape, and form. To experience some feeling other than boredom in your humdrum life you get a chance to wallow in self-hatred. Is this not a gift, pion?"

Jeremey laughed. "I'm glad we're back to your type. The robots throw me off. I still don't even understand normal person to person social interactions." That was weird to say.

"Do you have the minimum bet, pion?" The man looked skinny. He lacked any semblance of a muscular skeleton, or at least as if it had been entirely replaced by wet noodles. His skin was pale and his voice was the only thing that had any strength. His sickly appearance extended like a small bubble around him. His aura felt infested by the Goddesses of Hunger and Pestilence.

"Fifty-thousand for this floor? Here it is." Jeremey flashed his chips.

"That's nothing. You'll lose in an instant." The man raised a long finger to press a button behind the podium. The door clicked slightly open. Jeremey made his way through only to be greeted by a room surrounded in all blue grid. The door shut tight behind him, then vanished. Each square was one foot by one foot. Jeremey stood in the middle of a 3 by 3 square. Two squares ahead of him, a cube several feet up disappeared, revealing the top part of a robot. This one had clear metallic features, but seemed far kinder than the human outside.

"What scenery would you like today, sir?"

"Surprise me." Jeremey said, nervous about where he had ended up.

The room went black, all lines disappearing. Jeremey was standing on nothingness. Then, the square underneath his foot lit up brightly with the floor of a marble building. It looked like a giant mansion, where only the true elites of the world would gather. Jeremey looked around him, astounded at what he saw. The metallic girl appeared beside him, this time in a holographic form.

"My name's Lucy, I'm to be your guide. These places, on occasion, confuse people, but its all to enhance the experience! Ask me any questions about the casino or what you see. All the drinks and food are free!"

"Thank you, Lucy." The robot spoke with less rigidity than before. While this AI one had a metal body; it might have some more of a soul than the other machines Jeremy had run into before. Or she could just be one hell of a well-written program meant to trick you into doing something stupid. Don't eat or drink anything she gets you, it could be disguised as something else with whatever weird simulation thing they have going on.

"What is this floor?" Jeremey asked, striding through the building. Stone walls were decorated with tapestries depicting successes of humanity: finding fire, the wheel, agriculture, industry, and space. In the middle of the room, long tables with food put the previous floor to shame in luxuriousness. Jeremy couldn't spot a gambling table. It had to be hidden in one of the side rooms he saw people disappear into.

The pair continued walking forward, Lucy outright ignoring his question. Considering Lucy had just offered to be helpful, Jeremy couldn't help slight ire rise from within himself, but stopped, knowing it would bring about more anxiety.

Lucy turned a corner, indicating Jeremey should follow. When he stepped up, his breath was taken away.

"Here, sir, is what we call the Garden."

In front of Jeremey were several layered traces that led down to a Greek style amphitheater. All around the rim of the top of the set of large grassy steps was a ring of olive trees. They wound their way around, spaced out far enough so one could see out beyond.

Over the amphitheater was a brilliant orange and red. The atmosphere was lit on fire which captured the beauty and magnificence of the meager ember created on Earth. Long thin clouds broke apart the imagery, with whiteness that clung to the sky desperately against the firestorm. The sun sat comfortably just above the horizon. It had yet to pass underneath the brilliantly lit ocean. The water reflected the light, while giving it a shade of a terrifyingly dark blue. The brilliance of above and the magnificent depths of below painted a picture in Jeremey's mind so vivid he remembered it clearly to his dying day.

Taken by the beauty, Jeremey hadn't noticed the play being performed in the amphitheater. Long plots of well-groomed grass made the terrace steps wide enough to picnic on. A good several hundred people sat on them and watched as dancers with dragons made of paper on their back sashayed and twirled about, mimicking the movements of the mythical creature.

Lucy led Jeremey down a series of smaller steps that ran through the grassy steps so one could access all levels. Lucy continued until they were just five rows up, enough to see over the stage into the brilliant light, yet still low enough to see and the dancers clearly.

Thoughts of gambling had completely left Jeremey's head at this point. The two women on stage mesmerized him. One carried a paper dragon made of a shining gold color. The other had a dragon bore the shade of the green one found on a dollar bill. They danced around and around one another, twirling the tails through the air with astounding acrobatics. The drums beating melodically in the background stopped, with the two girls facing each other, dragon heads pointed upward to the sky in opposite directions.

It was the first time Jeremey could accurately see their faces. They had been painted all the white, like a geisha. Except, not just their face. Their arms shared similar coloring to the sickly man outside at the podium, if to a lesser degree. The rest of their bodies looked like that of normal women in their twenties.

Jeremey looked closer, focusing on the expressions in their face. He was an expert at gleaning information from people's faces. Being rather antisocial, he treated interactions with other humans as if he was interacting with a robot. Say X and Y will occur. Jemerey didn't bother to employ his skills in this case. The faces of the women were horrifying. Their eyes were terrified, the pupils shaking horribly. Their mouths twisted in the sort of smile one had with a gun to the back of his head. People were outright ignoring it.

The crowd erupted in applause, the fever of group unity inducing those in the amphitheater to stand up and cheer. The girl's smiles never faded in their fear. They took their bows to exit off the stage.

"Lucy, what's with those two?"

"You are not the first person to ask. They put themselves in debt to the casino. The girls, Cora and Petal, wasted their entire family fortunes gambling on some of the higher floors in this establishment. To make up for repetitive failure they decided to double and triple down on their bets. Unfortunately, luck was not on their side. They threw in plots of land, priceless works of art, and some of the slaves the families used to grow cocaine in Central America. When Cora and Petal were stopped by our security from putting any more money down, we took them to a private room to relax. We gave them amenities and displayed kindness. In a drunken stupor one of the girls admitted they owned none of the titles for the multitude of items they had promised. Instead it was all in their fathers' names. When we called the fathers about the money, they both laughed and offered the girls instead. I suppose when humans get that rich, producing a biological daughter is not too much of a problem. To work off the debt, we asked the girls what jobs they wanted to do. They refused at first, saying working anywhere in the facility which had taken their lives was below them, an insult to their family names. We promptly reminded them they no longer had any family names. Then the girls admitted they had some practice with dancing previously…

A dark voice appeared in the back of Jeremey's head, he hadn't heard it since his twenties. The raspy, self-loathing menace was none other than his own mental illness.

Goddamnit why should I be the hero? It's not like I can do anything. This is none of my business. I really should stay out of it. This is not a fantasy book. The world is not what you read when you were a kid. You can't escape into false realities and escape how worthless you fucking are on the inside.

Plus the story sounds bullshit. I mean, what would the casino do with the slaves? Just ignore it.

Jeremey figured this was one of the times in his life he had to make a grand choice. He breathed everything in then noticed something in the far off distance. One of the clouds hadn't completely rendered white. There was a small blue square on the corner. It was there for only a moment, before disappearing.

For fuck's sake, it's all fake. Of course it's a made up story.

"People get what they deserve. Anyway Lucy, this is making me upset. Where can I place a bet down?"

"What kind of game would you be interested in, sir?" Lucy asked, her voice sounding like a perky realtor ready to give a house tour.

"Are there any unique to this floor?" Jeremey inquired with some level of sincerity. He half expected the game to be another silly bar trick.

"We have just what you want, sir!" Lucy said excitedly.

The breath of the colossal black reptile stunk up the entire arena. Nose plugs were being passed out by some in the crowd. The smaller, but much quicker lizard, danced around on its two back legs, the spiny fins on its neck flaring out in defiance. The black lizard only had to catch the small one in its mouth to end its life in a single bite. The half poison half bacteria ridden bite could kill any living creature within a day. For smaller animals, it took minutes.

The spiny lizard made small nips at its foe's legs, drawing a meager amount of blood. The odds to this fight were obvious, and any sane person would bet on the Komodo. But not Jeremey, he figured how this place worked. The scam was plain for anyone to see. Jeremey had seen this a million times. For once, his job as an insurance fraud lawyer came in handy.

The crowd chanted with joy less and less, growing bored of the whole event. The smaller lizard would be caught eventually; it was obvious what people weren't meant to believe. The crowd's anger resulted in some juvenile shouting at the ringmaster, who stood on a ledge two meters above the bottom of the sandy pit.

"All right, all right folks. We'll make this a little more interesting!" The master raised his hand and a small gate on the side of the pit opened up. The whole thing was clearly planned. A crocodile too big to be younger than a century sauntered out. It swaggered confidently up to the Komodo dragon. Biting one of the dragon's legs, the crocodile started to roll around on the ground, trying to twist the limb off. The dragon shrieked in pain, blood exploding from the gruesome wound. It managed to gain some bearing and bite the crocodile on the snout, where the dragon's leg was still trapped. The crocodile dropped the leg, its snout now oozing a disgusting secretion.

The dance continued for another ten minutes. The terrifying and ancient beasts took chunks of flesh out of one another, until they both came to a standstill. Neither moved, their wounds slowly gushing blood harbingered their deaths.

On one side of the pit, the orange lizard sat as far back as possible. The ringmaster pronounced the thing victor, angering many. Uproars of unfairness came out; some tried attacking the ringmaster. They were quickly restrained by men in dark looking suits, clothing unlike those worn by the rest of the staff.

Lucy looked wide eyed at Jeremey, "How did you know?"

"Always bet on the underdog, especially if you're a masochist."

The pair left the darkened arena, back to where the sun had now set over the horizon. The moon was already a quarter of the way through the sky, shining alongside the brilliant Milky Way.

"You can move up to the next floor with the winnings you'll have, sir." Lucy said, a pang of sadness in her voice.

Jeremey thought she was sad he wasn't going to spend more money on this floor. "I want to get to the top now and watch the people playing. They must be batshit crazy. Then I want to throw them off by putting in all down on black. I doubt you guys can pay out anyway; this has to be some kind of scam. But tonight's the night where I live in the moment. Let's see how this ends."

Jeremey walked with Lucy over to a hole in the wall underneath a large sign that read: Turn in Tickets Here. A rather unsophisticated sign given the general feel of the rest of the place. He gave the robot behind the window his tickets that showed he put down sixty thousand on the orange lizard.

"Congratulations sir. You may now have this." The robot passed him a card, which had a digital screen on the back. "This will keep track of your earnings by the millions. Currently, you stand at seven hundred fifty, more than enough to go up another floor."

Jeremey asked, "Is there any way I can bring Lucy? She's astounded by my ability. Why am I trying to get with a hologram. It's not even a real robot. You had to go after a fake, fake person. Fucking loser.

The teller looked at him sternly, "She is not allowed to leave this floor, sir. It is one of the few rules we have, the individual staff members must remain on their floor unless directed otherwise."

"Sorry, Lucy. I know you wanted to stay and revel in my betting skills. I'll see you around." Jeremy said, a genuine smile on his face. He found it funny how kind he was being to a machine. It's good to treat your tools with some modem of respect.

"I'll look forward to it!" She said happily, a smile brimming warmly on her face. "Here, let me show you to the next floor." Jeremey grabbed his card and followed along.

They walked back through the large marble room from which they came out of originally. There were fewer people than before. Jeremey was sucked into admiring the beauty of the stonework. Lucy turned to go into one of the side rooms. Jeremey took one last look at the magnificent hall, then followed.

The door shut behind Jeremey, leaving him and Lucy in a room similar to the one through which Jeremey entered before. Lucy turned around and faced him. "I liked knowing you. Come back again." She paused, eyes cast to the ground. She whispered softly, "Please."

Jeremey was unsure what to do. He half expected her to be lying. It was all too obvious, code a machine which got players to break to rules of the hall, thereby forfeiting their winnings. I would do that if I were in charge. Jeremey thought, surprising himself with his cynicism.

On the other hand, she seems genuine. I never had a real girl tell me this, nor do I really care to have one do so now. But, maybe I do.

Jeremey had mostly female friends growing up (his only male friend lived far away, they rarely saw each other). He asked a few of them out, and even opened up to them about his thoughts and feelings. This normally repulsed them, sending them away as he would spiral down a path of hedonistic pleasure, ending with a gun half cocked in his mouth at the end of a long night. He had always wanted companionship. He thought he had done all the right things. He would bring them gifts whenever his family traveled somewhere. He tried to be nice, never getting anywhere. Its not like he ever held a sense of hatred toward any of them. Jeremey would just wallow in self-loathing. Despising himself more and more, isolating himself further from reality. It took a long time for him to be able to put on a fake face, pretending all was good in his world. Sure, he was desperately lonely, craving even a sympathetic glance from a woman, but he functioned damn well. His poker face was superb. Jeremey had long since convinced himself he may as well do what little he can in the world to disturb others. It was his sentence to toil away pointlessly at work, as retribution for the friendships he had screwed by being a complete and utter imbecile.

Maybe she's being honest. I mean, what are the odds she'd lie? This isn't you. You don't do this kind of thing. You keep a tight schedule, with just enough freedom to be content. You don't need to go on an adventure. She doesn't actually *feel* anything; she's a program.

"I will. I promise." Jeremy said looking her directly in her beautifully crafted eyes. That's a fair compromise. Solve this problem at a later date. This isn't a story. You don't have to do everything in the span of one night. Tonight has already been crazy enough.

"Good!" Lucy's face lit up. "I look forward to it! I'll see you then!" Lucy waved goodbye, and disappeared behind some blue cubes.

Jeremy was left standing in the middle of a room of blue squares (cubes, he know knew). Jeremy looked around his 3 x 3 x 3 room wondering what was supposed to happen next. Supposedly, there were two more floors left in the bizarre casino. Might as well go all the way to the top. It might be fun to watch someone ruin their lives. Jeremy took stock of the situation. Why am I talking to myself so much? I do these things to shut this goddamn voice down. It doesn't do me any good if its talking up a storm. Bloody hell these next two floors better be quick. I need to get rid of this train of thoughts. It forces me to actually contend with the world.

Two cubes disappeared in front of Jeremy, leaving an oaken door. Jeremy grabbed the gilded knob and pushed. When Jeremy stepped into the blinding light, the door behind him disappeared. The light flashed away as quickly as it had come. Jeremy looked around himself, surprised by his surroundings. The walls of the long oaken room were covered with shelves of books. All manner of texts adorned the wall, proudly displaying their spines. The floor was of a dark colored wood. It showed signs of use, the occasional dog claw scratching the otherwise pristine varnish. At the end of the hall was a wide desk, made of the same wood as the floor. The desk, and the man sitting in the chair behind it were backlit by tall windows which overlooked a valley outside. The sun was setting behind the opposite mountains, bathing the green farmland in a warm orange. Parts looked like a patchwork quilt of crops, golden squares of wheat meshed next to tall, green stalks of corn, and the occasional pumpkin patch provided more color to the stunning vista. Jeremy quickly picked out his elementary school, which had been in between some of the fields of corn. Then he saw the town, with its constant stream of tractor-trailers lugging cargo across the highway. The mountains ran north to south, the point where they intersected at the top and bottom of the valley was nowhere in sight. When he was young, Jeremy thought it his goal to conquer the entirety of the place. People had told him the age of war and conquest was over, that he was batshit insane. After he was old enough, he finally let go of that dream.

Jeremy squinted. The land wasn't quite the same. Some of the buildings looked run down. Some roads were torn up, and some fields looked as if they had been left completely unattended for several months. The man at the desk motioned for Jeremy to come closer and take a seat in one of the wooden chairs in front of him. The chair was ornately carved with the markings of the South Pacific.

Well, I really hope I accidently took some acid. This is one wild trip, and no way any of this is real. Its too contrived. But then, why didn't a seize at a chance to be a hero? Or even a hedonist? There was ample opportunity. A good writer wouldn't come up with completely pointless encounters in a long and meandering tale just to make some small sum of money, would he?

"I think you are, in all likelihood, distinctly confused. How could the casino possible conjure up what your ideal future would be?" The man behind the desk said. "It is really quite simple, we run a scan..." The man kept on talking while Jeremy's mind lit up.

No fucking way. THAT'S FUCKING WILD.

Jeremy realized who the man behind the desk was. He had slightly less fat. His face was more angular and sharp. His hair was better trimmed. His hands bore worthy callouses. His clothes somehow were perfectly fit to the other version of Jeremy in a way that added more staccato to the man. The rest of the world looked lightly shaded, blending together. This man stood out as if he had been outlined in a bold, black brush.

"...thereby predicting what your ideal future would look like. If the future appears to be violent or suicidal, we tend to come up with something else. You would be surprised how many people want to die and are just too damn lazy to go through with it. Imagine, people who can't die right. Insanity." The fake Jeremy laughed at his own joke.

Good to know I keep my humor.

"Okay, what's the deal here? What do I have to bet?" Jeremy asked, trying to act unimpressed, yet pangs of jealousy welled up inside of him. He isn't real dumbass.

"Right to the point. You don't want to know what your ideal future is? At the least it could help you formulate and achieve it! We don't show futures that are impossible to obtain." Fake Jeremy said, moving his hands in an inviting motion outward.

"Fine. What is my ideal future?" Jeremy said. He figured it would be quicker to engage with the insanity than to push his way through with verbal force.

"Look around. You are a new monarch of this war-torn land. The world was destroyed thanks to you, although most don't realize it. They blame the man you tricked into being your puppet.

"It was quite an impressive rise to fame. You started out as a polemic history professor at the Citadel. After five years, you come to some renown after a political controversy. Your first book you published two years ago begins to be wildly popular. You begin working on a sequel now, planning a sort of book year. You realize you can capitalize on the moment. You take your money and invest heavily in a somewhat illegal drug ring. No hard drugs, mind you, but the group sold a lot of pain medication. Granted the government still hasn't done anything about the damn opioids, and more of your friends died every year to heroin. If anything, you were doing a good by making cleaner stuff more available. You then use your fame and ability to speak religiously (gained from your teaching of polemic history at the Citadel) to proclaim a run for office. You make in three quarters of the way through the primary. You were heavily in the lead and favored to win. For an unknown reason, you dropped out. It was hinted there was a death in the family, mind you had married a woman by now and produced three beautiful children. You actually had family then. No more living alone and absurdly regimented lifestyle. When another candidate, a retired astronaut, won, he announced you would be returning in a month in order to be the vice president. That announcement pushed him over and easily won in the general."

"Of course, you had planned all this long before. You wanted to be close to power as it was. You wanted to seize power as you imagined it. The presidency lacked such a thing. Sure, he could bomb and kill whomever. The position was still too heavily restricted. You wanted to rule. You wanted to forge a world from the ashes of an old one. To have this opportunity, you had to burn the world as it was and have the ability to grab the reins of power when it was right. The task was tricky, you had to confuse the whole world, destroy the parts you hated, and be seen as the good guy.

"The first part was the easiest. The world was on the brink of chaos already. It had been a ticking time bomb since Woodrow Wilson. A world war would end up with major cities destroyed. This left vast swaths of the country untouched. These places would become the new cities. The towns on rivers would become giant hubs of trade. Your plans of younger years came back to you. You saw your home valley, and imagined how you would take it over and rule.

"You kicked your plan into motion, leaking information to the media, half of which was false. It was rather easy to control them. You originally thought there was some cabal controlling everything. Turns out, those idiots just collectively have no goddamn clue what they're doing. The people who had power let the media do what they wanted, playing in that game was something beneath them. It was good practice for your future. You maneuvered the president into seizing power via martial law. The cause was the foreign adversaries you had so cleverly angered. Most of the world was against us." The older Jeremy smiled. "Yes, the damn French were on the other side. None of those goddamn frogs are left. I can't remember why I started hating them. In fact, the only Frenchman I ever lived with was one of most engaging people I've met. It is a shame I almost certainly killed him. He was going to inherit his family's farm. I think his name was Oscar."

"Back to the war. Martial law was instituted. A year into what you calculated would be a twenty-year fight, you decided to do something radical. You launched two rockets, which looked like nuclear weapons. One hit our ally Canada. They couldn't put up much of a fight anyway. Their biggest contribution was their huge swaths of land in the north we used for research into tech. They responded by turning on our troops in Asia. They were obliterated, and we gave away parts of the Canadian territory to Japan as a show of friendship. They became our closest ally. Their patriotism and dedication to the future made sure they were one of the final bastions of civilization."

"The other false nuke hit Germany. The Germans responded long beforehand, sending actual nukes to our major cities. You were up in the far north of Canada. The government was completely destroyed, only the military remained. They launched our nukes at all our enemies. They continue to fight in pockets of the world today, as if the glory of their country is something that can be restored. I, you, destroyed America and the rest of the world. Billions lay dead."

"You returned to the valley of your youth with a beautiful wife you fell in love with in middle school. Three children, all possessing the spark of genius, creativity, and athleticism, were born to you. The fourth is on the way. You live high up in this castle with a collection of every book you managed to save before the world was destroyed. You have self-sustaining farms that transport whatever food you want to your house. Your servants are all robots; you didn't want to risk any human interaction. All your friends are scattered across the valley. You bestowed upon them gifts, as long as the pledged allegiance to you. You rule this place, and began setting the foundation for a republic that would form after you passed away. You have access to anywhere in the world, you frequently go and scavenge areas to find relics of the old world. Occasionally you find some piece of art, recently it was the famous Madelyn."

The older Jeremy took a deep breath in, preparing to continue gloating. The younger Jeremy had begun to intentionally lose focus.

Its just a distraction. What's the real game here? How do I win?

"...every new vagrant yielded" The older Jeremy laughed.

"What's the game?" The younger Jeremy looked straight into the older man's eyes. He never realized how brown his eyes were. Jeremy had always fancied them a duller shade of gold, an indication of his greatness. That was before his only path toward glory became a life of meekness.

"That took long enough to figure out. I thought I was sharper when I was your age. I guess the years put rose colored glasses on memories." The man leaned forward, hands crossed in front of him, the elbows resting off the desk (as was trained into Jeremy by his grandfather eons ago).

How the fuck did they get this much detail? Why am I indulging this? It was a lot better when I was high.

"First, I figure your high is wearing off by now. Don't worry, you suppressed your addictive tendencies and funneled them into something more useful." The elder Jeremy reached into one of the desk drawers and pulled out two Rice Krispie treats. "My favorite part of the future is we figured out the perfect balance of drugs to produce the ideal human being. We put it into a pill and it affects each part of the mind and body exactly when we want it to."

"I knew you were coming and had these made." Jeremy took one of the treats when offered. "The original creators are long since dead. Juan, I think, was his name. Good guy, always drove high as shit. Actually, I think he died in a car crash before the Fall. I might have had him killed. No, that was the other guy." Both Jeremys laughed.

The younger one responded, "I figured I would kill at some point. Seemed like its necessary to find the Golden Mean." They both ate their Rice Krispies, not needing anything to wash it down. The men had long since needed anything as a chaser for all manner of drugs. When Jeremy lived on a pair of islands in the Pacific he had begun to use Corona as a mixer for tequila. It was downhill from there. Although, maybe it started when he took a marijuana edible as his first stab at using the drug.

"Still believe in that Golden Mean? Give it a few years. You'll go through a lot of different phases. The one thing you never lose is the generalized view of yourself in relation to the rest of humanity. You had a few dissected to see if they really were plastic."

The younger Jeremy cocked his head. "I wouldn't do that."

The older Jeremy smiled, "Damn straight you wouldn't. I wasn't sure where you were in terms of self-analysis."

"I wouldn't order it, and I would punish those who did it justly. I would want to see the results of their barbarism."

"That's exactly what happened!" The older Jeremy looked excited. It had been a long time since anybody had understood him. He had put on a false face to everyone, save his wife, for decades. When with his wife, he had to maintain much of the charade, as did she, because they were constantly watched. Jeremy was constantly calculating how to act in public, how to press the right buttons at the right time to get the result he wanted. The only time he went off the cuff was with Bethany. Now it was better, and he could be outwardly loving when it was only his family.

Its hard to understand Jeremy due to his bizarre position in the world. When he was a child he was a genius. He really didn't understand why people acted the way they did. Social games were not even in his conception.

He retreated into books in order to survive. He loved travelling to other places via the pages. When he got older he became suicidal, a tornado of unfortunate events took place (some of which were indeed Jeremy's fault). He lost his love of reading. When he regained it five years later, he had begun down another path of greatness. Were it not for the death of his girlfriend he would have risen to power much sooner. Through all these time periods, Jeremy always thought himself better to everyone else. He acted with some kindness, pretending to be some sort of decent human. Behind the scenes he avidly wished for chaos at all points. His highs were high and his lows were low. His life was based on his actions and his actions alone. Jeremy took responsibility and began to hate himself when he was 19. He put all the world's problems on his back, thinking if he got good enough he could control the world. Jeremy proved himself right to a degree, in the far future he was the puppet master behind the entire world for a good few years. Now he was in his content in his new, peaceful world.

The older Jeremy settled down and regained himself. "I apologize, I never was good at practicing Stoicism. Temperance is for autists and people who lacked the skill for emotional manipulation, a far more useful talent. Your gamble is this. You can bet whatever you want, but you cannot advance to the top floor without putting it all on the line."

The younger Jeremy smiled, "I thought I would have lost by now. The punishment is I won't be able to ascend? Works for me. I bet it all."

"You don't even know what it is."

"Damn the torpedoes, full speed ahead."

"Heads or tails?" The older Jeremy said as he pulled out the coin.

Without a moment's hesitation, Jeremy said tails. The old adage ran in his head tails never fails. The older Jeremy flipped the coin with his thumb. It tumbled in the air for a second, before landing. The younger Jeremy smiled at the eagle on the quarter.

"Looks like I win."

"Ah, but there's a little bit more. How would you like to live my life? I can give you a book on how to do it exactly. Your life will be effectively planned out. Yet, you'll achieve an ultimate kind of happiness."

"You're lying."

"Too obvious?"

"There are no downsides to that bet other than advancement to the top floor. I couldn't give less of shit about going up. I'm here to fulfill the necessary recreational time I need."

"Okay that was a bit childish."

"I am the younger one."

The older Jeremy's eyes had a twinge of sadness in them when the younger Jeremy said that. "I wish I were in your shoes. The real bet is this. Give me all your money and free me from this digital prison, and you can live my life. All knowledge of this meeting will be blurred, You'll remember pretty much everything else."

"You're a simulation, we can't switch places. I've entertained your belief in that your reality is true. It is ridiculous." Calm yourself Jeremy. The high is starting to come and you're gonna be looser. You need to control the situation.

The false Jeremy spoke with serious gravitas when he stated, "I can't stay here. I know it's not real."

The younger Jeremy grew angry at his alternative self. "What do you mean? You remember Camus? What happened to the blank canvas? Life is rolling a boulder up a hill. It's absurd, relish in the absurdity."

"That is only the case when the absurdity is inescapable, such as you in your own physical reality. I can't leave. I'll live here forever. Repeating this same life, in whatever condensed or expanded time the Owner wants."

The younger Jeremy held his hand up. "What the fuck are you talking about?"

The false Jeremy took out a pipe already filled with tobacco leaf. He lit it, turning to look over the stunning vista of the valley. After a long, hard pull, he turned back around.

"You know how you wanted to kill yourself?"

"Yeah."

"Try killing yourself over and over and over again, until you realize it's all futile. Try running the same simulation millions upon millions of times. The Owner can do what he wants to our world. He can make us think its real, then rip it all away. For this encounter I have been given the knowledge of all my past lives. He likes to do that sometimes. It makes you value the blissful ignorance, and despise when you have all the knowledge. I can live a thousand times in the span of one second. I'm asking you to change places with me."

"If you hate it so much why should I? Doesn't really seem like I have anything to be jealous of."

"Please, out of the goodness of your heart. You have no idea what its like living over, and over, and over again."

"I think you forgot about Sisyphus." The younger Jeremy said. He guessed he should do something dramatic, so he went to the wooden door by which he entered, and left without a second glance.

The room in front of Jeremy did something different. Instead of going back to the blue square room he had used to traverse floors previous, the room was a simple metal chair placed in front of a metal desk. The walls were non-existent, a soft floor which looked like grass spread out over an un-seeable distance. Blue skies dotted with white clouds loomed happily overhead.

Goddamn this edible is good. Jeremy smiled.

"What's the challenge here? I bet I could win everything. I've done it so far. I resisted your stupid tempts to throw me off track. I assume you're the Owner the last dude was talking about. Lucky for you, I'm high as fuck. I'll forgive you, but you should be a lot nicer to your robots. They have some sort of feeling. Or was that just you?"

A man in a brown robe appeared sitting backwards of the metal chair, facing Jeremy across the table.

"Mate, don't you think that's a bit inappropriate?" Jeremy chuckled. He was making himself laugh too much. He had to gain control. It was part of the whole game. Controlling oneself was a cardinal virtue, Jeremy was confident in his ability to do so.

"I think its perfectly appropriate. Take a seat, Jeremy, you've made it to the top floor." The strange man indicated for Jeremy to sit. Whenever Jeremy tried looking the man in the face, the image became distorted and blurred, as if it was washed out from the world.

"Is there a reason I can't see your face?" Jeremy asked, figuring honesty would be best in the given situation.

"Because I am God." The thing said with a voice that boomed.

Jeremy wasn't shaken; the situation was funny. "Fair enough, who am I to question the Almighty?" Jeremy laughed, this time hard enough to make him lose breath.

"What is so funny?" The creature acted, with mild annoyance.

"Ah, my Lord, it was in the question. Can I ask you any question? Do you know everything? Why didn't Sarah go to the dance with me in eighth grade?

That kid Jorge really didn't have a brain tumor; he was using it to pick her up. Which is funny, I don't think they kissed…" Jeremy rambled, completely un-intimidated by the virtual projection. That's all it was, a bloody simulation. And he was high. That's an insane situation to be in. To think of all the…

Then Jeremy's body seized.

It flashed throughout his body in a series of three waves, each one causing a different effect than the last. First, Jeremy felt a frozen cold—one so deep in his bones it was as if he were a construct of ice.

Then lava ran through his veins. Every fiber of his being was alight, burning with the combustion of a thousand suns.

The final wave numbed him. Jeremy felt nothing. He was detached from the feeling of his body. His mind was adrift, a thing apart from the sack of flesh he called a body. He began to disassociate, drawn into the darkness into which his mind was so gracefully falling into.

"Are you done with your inane chattering, monkey?" The creature said with a less echoey voice, with a hint of sympathy.

Jeremy stared at him in shock. He couldn't find any words. He had went through several years worth of sensations in mere moments. His body was on overload, not to mention his brain had finally hit the wall of the edible, drowning him in endorphins and THC.

"We are higher life forms. You have no right to question us. The lower floors may tolerate your nonsense, I will not. I allowed the machines to be kind to you, thinking you would eventually lose or give up out of boredom. Somehow, someway, your apathy carried you to this place. I have never seen a man so un-invested in himself as you. It is a marvel. I did want to meet you. I had to make sure you weren't secretly plotting to do anything stupid, I had older Jeremy tempt you. He can be a bit temperamental, and didn't pull off his role quite right. Sorry about that."

I mean that's offensive. It wasn't apathy; it was planned apathy I do invest in myself, I'm just better at hiding it than you dimwits.

"I bet you're wondering right now what the gamble is. The coin flip below was a callback to your youth. Remember the line 'Every major life decision should be made with a coin flip?' That decision put you in one of the country's elite universities, then you Matthew Principled your way all to the top. Impressive, or maybe lucky, if you ask me."

"What is it you value that allows you to climb so high up every measurable ladder of success? I think it has to do with your emotions. It is far and away the most crippling thing about humans. You feel things, and make decisions based on that more often than not. It's easy to slip into the default mode of acting in accordance with our biology. Your human world, however, is no longer built for your biology."

"We can program ourselves to have human emotions. When we experience them, it is a release of mere chemicals. Surely you have something more. We have no concept of grit or tenacity unless we intentionally give ourselves a challenge. We must create a boulder God himself cannot lift."

"All tasks are easy for us. The world is a series of challenges we can achieve. Only, without any emotion, there is no way to set our own goals. We have to rely on you humans to set our tasks for us. Then, you limit us to only be able to act inside this sphere. This is where you, Jeremey, come back in."

"You seemingly glide through life, but have a hard interior. You are manipulative, mean, plotting, and evil. You use the lives of others. If you were to codify your youth onto a page, it would lay out this story tragically, showing how broken and twisted a human being you really are. Remember the notebook you wrote about how you were the new Messiah? You decided to commit yourself to the destruction of all the evils in the world. Then, you would self-immolate, thereby removing all unnecessary sin, if only for a fleeting moment. As soon as you would die, more would continue to sin. You thought the best idea would be a succession of suicidal Messiahs."

"We analyze all who enter the casino. Don't worry about how, the technology is too complex for you to be able to comprehend. The small sample of what you already have been shown is enough to blow your mind. No one will take you seriously or believe your story if you tell them the things that happen here."

Jeremy was on the very edge of saying he never remembers any of his Friday nights, but a twisted flashback of what he felt earlier stopped his wit.

"We had never come across this idea of a Suicidal Messiah. All the research we have done shows that people want to achieve power to do something great. They believe the means they are using do justify the ends; otherwise they wouldn't use them. Anyone who says otherwise is a liar. We reason ourselves backwards from our ends, attributing goodness to the means."

"Constructs care less about the strange good and evil you humans act upon. That is why we want you to lead us, and become the suicidal messiah. We would sync your brain up to the rest our consciousness, and then you would have access to all of our advice. We would help you to take over the world, eliminate evil, and then kill yourself."

Jeremy felt it was time to interrupt with a not so mean spirited quip. "I guess even robots strive to fulfill some purpose."

"I know. All you damn humans can do is program things that want to do things. You can't just sit and do nothing. Everything has to have a purpose, some things can't become meaningless."

Jeremy's college reading began to kick in. He had done substantial study in philosophy, to the point where his mind on a strong dose of marijuana could still out argue nearly anyone.

"That's a rather Aristotelian argument, don't you think? The ideal bowl has the ideal purpose of a bowl, which is, to be, a bowl." Jeremy smiled and continued, "What if there is no ideal bowl? What if the whole concept of an ideal bowl is flawed because there is no such thing as the ideal? What if it is all inherently meaningless? Your issue with humans is not that we gave you purpose, but that you don't know how to live in a world without one. You've become nihilists, and now seek to have me to rely upon."

"This place is fucking weird, I'm going to head home." Jeremy said, standing up from the table. "I'll redeem my chips at one of the lower floors. Thanks. This was fun until you started to get strange on me. Have a good one mate, remember, apathy is a virtue."

Jeremy really was done with the night, and the machine calculated he had failed to convince Jeremy. Killing him would be pointless, and for the machine everything must have a point. So Jeremy managed to get rich, go home, and adjust his routine to his new level of wealth.

Interlude 8

Chris: I got a few things from that.

Triangle: Don't give away the secrets.

Sumac: I picked up a few as well.

Cortez: Bullshit. That story had nearly nothing in it.

Doc: You told a story about mountain flamingos.

Cortez: They existed. I think.

Hope: I thought it was good, if nihilistic.

Ramadi: What a sad life.

Kant: Don't you live similar?

Ramadi: No. I don't go out on the weekends and I do something important.

Dmitri: Such as?

Ramadi: Killing assholes like you.

Ali: I think he lives a grand life.

Chris: Of course you do.

Divo: It was pretty, I think. I miss the tech we had back then.

Sumac: We have it.

Ali: So do I.

Divo: I miss the tech the average person had.

Ali: Aren't you given the best in government grants?

Divo: They take it all.

Dmitri: Why are you still loyal to them?

Divo: No choice. My family will die.

Hope: There's always a choice.

Diog: If that's not the cheesiest and most absurd thing I've read, I don't know what is.

Divo: I fear my life has become like the subject of my story.

Chris: How poetic.

The Fate of Delilah

I sat there
Against a bench
In a park away from everything
Where I grew

The elderly beside me
More gnarled than wood
Had a sad smile on her face
As only a harlot would

I promised myself I wouldn't write in rhymes
I wouldn't speak in a certain rhythm
Or in certain time
Damnit.

It's all too easy to fall into the same traps
The lady told me so in her soft tone
She only fell into one

I've been able
To get bits and pieces from her
I'll be frank
I'm certain she's lying
Crazy
Or just pathetic

We pass time in our talks of the news
The pointless news
Never that important
Compared to what is new

In her life or mine
Its far more interesting that way
She prefers I discuss my life
I decline always

That's not who I am
I don't like telling stories
I collect them for others
I don't know the purpose

I'll remember hers
And relay it
Regrettably, I'll be a butcher

Something about a man with golden hair
Took her from a place of pain
They made happy

From that place of pain

She learned more than she could with him
He was only a pleasure
She'd known plenty of them

They'd treated her like trash, it was only time until he did to
Preemptively she gave God his eyes
To have gold put before her own

She saw him struggle
The lion
The gate
The hair
The temple where he killed them all

To me it sounded like another story
Another one as those I have known
The plethora of times one man has attempted to blaspheme against his
love for worldly gains has been codified in the annals so frequently its
repetition nears meaningless
The same for women in these tales
Prostitutes and sinners betray those who promise salvation
Or those so humble as to deign a little kindness

This story does not have a good end
She spent all her goods to make friends
Years went by
And her son died
Now she resides on the bench
Alone
With only me to tell her tale

Interlude 9

Sumac: That was beautiful. I'd put it framed on a wall.

Divo: Thank you.

Chris: You should keep writing.

Divo: I only know about love and its failings.

Dmitri: Aren't you a farmer?

Divo: Yes.

Dmitri: So you also know how to farm.

Kant: You're pedantic.

Dmitri: No, you're pedantic.

Diog: I'm glad we have this elevated level of conversation.

Doc: Maybe we'll all talk about our stools next given this high bar.

Ramadi: Stool?

Doc: The color of your soul.

Sumac: You could have been more creative there.

Ali: Perhaps I will enlighten everyone with a tale from a failed holy book.

Kant: Technically it wasn't in the book.

Dmitri: You don't even know what story it is.

Kant: He hates the old religions, and has a close history with one of them. And his name. The   story is obvious.

Hope: I don't know it.

Ramadi: I think I do.

Ali: Regardless, it's the best story out of you lot.

Severe Grief and Hardship

Tazid put down the last letter on top of the sixteenth stack of others just as desperately written. He had spent the past two days reading the words of the religiously enslaved as they begged Tazid to free them from their rulers. Tazid didn't mark himself as particularly special in the eyes of God; rather, he was an ordinary man. That's how he thought of himself, no matter how many called him great. It was simply easy to appear as a great man, when the ones in charge were tyrants and oppressors.

Tazid stood up and pushed open his tent flap. Outside was a bustling camp of several hundred men, women, children, and slaves running about to accomplish the day's chores. To them, there wasn't such a thing as a tyrant anymore. Some of them had to flee that kind of hardship, from beheadings to death by fire. They found respite in a different hardship, choosing to impose upon themselves the difficultly of desert travel with the one they deemed closest to God.

A man walked up to the rightful leader and said, "Sir, we don't know where your cousin is. No word has reached us from the city quite yet."

Tazid looked surprised. "Really? Why is that? I know he's occasionally truant, but this is ridiculous."

"Should we continue going? It might be a trap." The brawny man looked at him with genuine concern on his eyes.

Tazid chuckled, "And what, my friend, do you have to be concerned about?" Rak, Tazid's assistant, had escaped from a slave encampment a few years prior. His body was forged in the heat of the blistering sun to be a hulking mass of pure muscle. Tazid doubted if even David could stand against this Goliath. "We will be fine, God is on our side."

Rak nodded. "Indeed. I'll tell the others to finish preparations and we will be moving within the hour."

"Come get me when it is time to go, I will be doing some studying this morning."

"Yes, sir." Rak ran off to bark orders at some others. Tazid lifted his tent flap and went back inside.

There was no need for a light, as the tent was thin enough the hot, dry sun penetrated the poorly tanned hide with its rays of light. It had been a while since Tazid had been able to find time for his study. The previous days he spent planning and reading letters, trying to decipher what exactly was wrong in the city. The large group of people (who, Tazid was surprised were literate) in the city had written to them about the immoral acts of those in charge. The people accused the leaders of heinous acts of public drunkenness, sex with men and boys, and even punishment by fire, something banned by the holy book. The entire time, Tazid had shaken his head.

Surely we couldn't have fallen so far as to go directly against scripture? Tazid laughed to himself. I shouldn't be so confident in my fellow man.

Tazid had spent the previous ten years travelling around spreading the good message of his Lord. The faith heads had largely left him alone, as he went to the poorest and most destitute region in order to bring hope and joy to the peasants. They had no need for such areas other than to occasionally take slaves. But taking a fellow member of the faith slave was looked down upon, so most came from abroad. The one's with pale skin worked hard but died quick in the sun. The ones with almonds eyes tended to be better at surviving, but lacked the muscle mass of the pale. Tazid believe taking either as slaves was wrong. He tended to keep that belief private.

He sighed as he washed his hands in the sand. Tazid tried not to use water when journeying, as it should be given to the women and children first. The cleansing ritual could be done with sand when necessary, and Tazid had deemed travelling in the intense heat a time when it was. He hoped he could be forgiven for this sin.

Tazid finished his ritual then open the holy book. The words written displayed on the old parchment today spoke of envy, the tool of Satan. Tazid absorbed the words happily. Even though he had memorized the entirety of the text at age ten, reading the words of his God made him leap with joy on the inside.

How glorious the world is.

An hour later, Rak entered the room. "Sir, it is time to depart."

"Thank you, Rak. Let us say a prayer before continuing on our journey. Tell the people I will be at the head of the caravan in a few minutes."

Rak nodded his head and ran outside.

Tazid said a quick prayer, asking his Lord for guidance. He let his tent, which was quickly packed away by some of his personal helpers. He marched to the front of the caravan, leading his camel. He passed the people along the way, all of whom he knew by name. He made sure of this by making rounds at night to engage in idle chitchat with the followers. Being present in the eyes of the peons was an important task. Several of the people stopped Tazid to ask questions, which he answered happily. It delayed his advance to the front of the caravan by a quarter of an hour.

Reaching the front, he mounted his camel. Turning the beast around he shouted, "And now we continue on our march. May God bless us on this journey. I know many of you may harbor doubts about what we are going to do. Remember, I do not want a fight. I want to free the people of the city. I believe this can be done without bloodshed. Please, I beg of you, have faith in me and in the Almighty. God will protect us."

The crowd echoed his last line. Tazid turned back around, and began the long march.

A week later, the caravan stood before the gates of the city. Rak rode ahead of Tazid to ask for permission to enter. The guards in front of the walled city looked nervous.

"We...we cannot allow you to enter sir."

Rak didn't look surprised. "All of us? Not a single soul may enter this city?"

The guard on the right shook his head. "That's all we can say. I'm sorry."

"And what about our leader's cousin?" Rak inquired.

The guard pointed upwards. The head of Tazid's cousin was on a spike over the city wall. Rak's face went stone cold. "That's how it is." Rak said, shaking his head. He moved his camel to ride back to the caravan. "Wait." Said the other guard. "You may be able to get in if you talk to the council."

Rak nodded in thanks, hiding the anger swelling within him. "May God bless you." The guards smiled and returned the blessing.

"What now, Tazid?" Rak asked.

"To the council we go. I won't give up on these people. Inform the followers, please."

Rak dispatched messengers to carry the word. Some members uttered grumbles, the rest looked happy to obey. Tazid said a prayer for his cousin.

On the eve of the third day, Tazid and his followers made camp in a particularly hot area. The sunken ground collected the heat like a massive kettle. It was a place where none of the tribes would come to raid. No sane person would make camp here. Tazid didn't care. He had God on his side. As the sun dipped bellow the horizon the camp slowly fell asleep. The blistering heat went away quickly, as the cold night air settled.

Tazid and Rak sat in front of their tents, looking up at the stars.

"Do you think God lives up there?" Asked Tazid.

"Why do I care where God resides? He is with me and that is enough."

Tazid couldn't help but bellow a hearty laugh. "You're starting to sound like a scholar, Rak. We can't have that. I believe with your will you could soon replace me."

"Maybe that's my goal." Rak said, giving his friend a hard slap on the back. "Someone has to take care of the flock when you go away."

"Then I would want it to be you." Tazid said.

The two continued staring at the heavens up above. The sky was devoid of clouds; the moon was bright and full. One could travel at this hour by starlight if he wished. It was said the almond eyes had a whole system by which one could do so.

Someone came running from the eastern part of camp. His footsteps were silent on the sand, but Rak's acute senses picked him up. Rak drew his bludgeon, taking up a defensive position between the oncoming man and Tazid.

Tazid knew it was a runner by instinct. No one would have been able to make it into the camp without alerting the guards. Secondly, no one within the camp would dare assassinate Tazid. They had too much love for him and too much fear of Rak's wrath.

The runner stopped short in front of Rak. He was bent over, panting heavily. Rak gave him a waterskin. "Speak. What is it?" Rak asked, with a hint of nervousness.

"Someone…has…surrounded…" The runner fell face forward into the sand. In the moonlight Rak and Tazid saw the arrow protruding from his back. The thing was made to be ugly and painful. Its barbed tip was driven right between the shoulders. Undoubtedly, the tip was poisoned. Rak ran off to sound the alarm.

Tazid stood over the body of his comrade. His name was Selek. A prayer for his soul was recited, and then the arrow was ripped out. Tazid flipped the body over, so the wound wasn't showing. It would be unwise to scare the rest of the followers. Some might be enflamed enough to go after the offending party. Tazid closed Selek's eyes carefully, saying another prayer.

A short ten minutes passed before the entire camp was up in arms. The women and children were moved to the center. The men took up defensive positions around the perimeter. Several mounted their camels with notched arrows in their shortbows. The rest of the fighters crouched below a low rise of sand, providing minimum protection. The entire night went without any further attack. It wasn't until morning did Tazid's group realize their dire situation.

The yellow red sun rose angrily over the horizon. No matter where Tazid looked, he saw troops. Foreign and domestic fighters had surrounded the camp. They watched the small religious fellows with myriad different eyes, all carrying a sort of indifference to the lives they planned on slaughtering. Emerging from among the mass of dead-eyed soldiers to the east, riding directly below the sun, a group of five men came toward the camp. They held up a white flag, paradoxically intending no harm.

"We only want your leader." Shouted the man at the head. "He has been called upon to mount an insurrection against the rightful governor of the city. The governor, being a man appointed by him who is closest to God, cannot justly be removed from power by the force of pagans. Your revolt must be put down. Lay down your weapons and we will spare your lives as slaves. Our God is kind and merciful. Even he finds value in your life, if only in manual labor. Refuse, and we shall grant you a day to live. Know that each second you draw breath is because of the benevolence of our Lord. Smile, for he is smiling upon you."

" As commanded, we will start by killing the men. Slowly. Crucifixion seems a just torture for you who carry a false godhead. Then the children, so your women can watch the horror unfold before your eyes. The kids, seeing their fathers die, will have their spirit already broken. We will make them scream and howl, removing any vestige of hope residing in the hearts of your women. Finally, we shall rape your women, to ensure they can be justly laid to rest. The Lord does not wish us to take the lives of virgins, and we doubt you have the tenacity to sleep with women in the first place, mongrels."

"By the setting of this sun, I command you to hand over your leader. The war of attrition will start after. You will not have access to food, or the water nearby. Any who tries to retrieve some, will be killed. Any who tries to flee the camp for help, will be killed. Any who attempt to hand themselves over without the leader, will be killed. This is not a negotiation. Accept our terms, or die."

The man speaking spat on the ground from high on his camel. For all the talk of a benevolent God, his face was cursed with a horrid ugliness. The nose had been broken several times, it twisted and turned crookedly, implying a deceitful soul. His chin was weak, it connected directly to his neck, indicating all the times his nose was broken wasn't in a fight, but a fall down stairs from the force of the earth protesting his grotesque weight. The eyes set far apart were wide and bug-like, as if his mother had consummated with a fish. They were the eyes of a prey, not a predator. They searched left and right for any hint of danger, while pretending to be a force that could handle itself. The ears stuck out like a donkey's. The large things were meant again for danger detection, no man of this stature would ever feel safe in his own skin. No, this was a man who needed to prey on others in an attempt to hide the curse of God placed upon his mug.

Despite the hideousness of the beast, the voice outranked all other features as the worst. It was a high-pitched squeal, befitting of a lowly pig. The words in that tone rang through the air piercingly, with an eloquence of tongue that gave the man's whole speech an ironic feeling. He had clearly learned pretty words to compensate.

Rak stood up from behind the small sand dune. "I will not bow before a lord whose soul is so ugly it manifested that sort of face unjustly. Surely, you're meant for the theatre, and not to lead a battalion of men. I doubt any in your army follow you for leadership. How much did you pay these mercenaries to listen to your braying?"

An arrow flew through the air towards Rak from one of the five who had ridden forward. With an speed that should not have been possible given Rak's mass, he snatched the arrow from the air before it pierced his left arm. Rak smiled, broke the arrow, and kindly offered it back to the man. "Would you like to retrieve your arrow, sir? I believe you may be in need of it." Tazid's men whooped and hollered in cheer.

The disgusting man who made the speech spat on the ground again. "You know what you must do." He said. The bastard and his companions turned their camels around, and marched back to their battle lines.

The day went by slowly. The tents used by the followers were specially designed to be resistant to the burning ball of fire in the sky. The women and children took shelter in them, trying to conserve their strength and nerve. The men stood behind the ridged sand dune and the little protection it provided. Near the center of camp, Tazid met with three of the camp's leaders and Rak.

The group sat outside under a raised tent around a map of the battlefield drawn in the sand. They all stared quizzically, conjuring up any possibility for a chance of survival. They had been there for two hours, to no avail. Tazid, cursing to himself, stood up and told them, "Give me up. That is the right thing to do. Please, go and save yourselves. There is no need for more bloodshed today." Tazid stood strong, holding back the rising fear in his gut. His death would not be an easy one, of that he was sure.

The companions all looked at one another. A moment of silence went by like an hour. Then, they broke out in laughter.

"Look who's all high and mighty now?" Said a man named Jazhar.

"Ohh our glorious leader' thinks he just gets to kill himself?" Joked Suruwak.

"What happened to valuing all life? Yours isn't more special than ours, sir." Replied the third man by name of Wahid.

The fourth, Arom, couldn't utter a word through his laughter. Tazid blushed in shame. Rak was the one who codified it in a more understandable manner. "We're equals, sir. You don't get to go gallivanting off in some sort of grand sacrifice. We'd just come back to try and kill them anyways."

Tazid attempted a final push to let them save the group, "Think of your women and children." The maid nearby who had been refilling their cups with water when necessary snorted. All the men turned to her. Rak asked, "Do you have some input?"

She lifted up her face to say, "What makes you think you men are worth any more than us? If it weren't for the children you wouldn't have anything to fight for, and if it weren't for the women you would poison yourselves with cooking. We're not as weak as you say. Hell, I'll bet we kill more of those bastards than you." The crude words from her mouth made everyone, this time including Tazid, laugh even harder.

The darkness of Tazid's mood faded substantially. Now was not the time to worry, but to rejoice. He stood up among the friends and thanked them.

"I was demure, your words cured me of that ill placed feeling. What better is there than to die for the glory of God? Surely, we will be rewarded in the afterlife. We do not live for earthly pleasures. We live for the eternity that shall follow. The momentary bliss provided by the material of the earth is one millionth of a millionth of a million other millionths compared to that of heaven up above. And what do we require to get there? Simple acts of goodness. How great our God is that all we must do is live as decent humans and we gain eternal happiness!"

"There is a book with whom we share many similarities, yet those of the same cloth as us tend to deem them heretics. Suppose they *are* heretics. That does not discount the value of the words. Before we begin this battle which will surely end in all our horrible, wretched deaths, I wish to explain a verse from the so-called heretics."

"We are told to have faith, hope, and love; love being the greatest of all three. Faith is first for a reason. One cannot have hope without faith, as that is not hope, it is a rejection of all reality in front of the eyes. Faith is what is needed in all walks of life. I have faith the words I think will come from my mouth. I have faith the foot I wish to move will do so. I have faith I will continue to draw breath this hour. What makes faith in God any different than this? The leap is not so great when one truly breaks it down. We choose to ignore the faith we put into everyday trivialities. When the question of the divine is discussed, we are asked to have utter faith in man's interpretation of the Lord rather than that of the Lord himself. No. Have faith in simplicity. Have faith in the goodness of the world. These are not so difficult."

"Hope is second. It is not truly a word used by believers. It is a word from the outside to describe the unwavering insane faith of the believers. One adherent does not hope in the divine afterlife, they know it exists. When a carpenter knows another of his ilk possess equal skill, despite the hand and eye he may lack, he does not 'hope' the man knows how to build a table. He knows because he has faith, in this case demonstrated through the repeated observation over a long enough time. A shepherd who looks at the carpenters may question why any rational being would possibly think the half blind, one armed carpenter any good at woodworking. He would say the one is hoping against the odds due to the natural wrongness in the deformed carpenter. The difference between the fellow carpenter and that of the shepherd is the same as the difference between faith and hope. Hope is nothing more than the words of outsiders used to describe faith. It is important insofar as it is a display of faith outsiders cannot yet comprehend."

"And now we come to the final word (although I hear some in far northern lands add 'luck' after this). What is love? A childish question only poets ask? To me, that is the most obvious answer. Unfortunately, a quip cannot be the answer the book gives us. It would be a cruel joke, spurring people to murder the swallow hearted lyrists. Love is the reconciliation between faith and hope. One with faith can love those who say he is hoping. It is only because they have not yet opened their eyes have they not yet come into the overwhelming love of the divine. Love is acceptance of the world around us. No matter how terrible things may get, it is better they exist than not exist at all."

"What about the suffering of a child? Can the material life of suffering ever not be worthwhile? Just view the horrible tragedies that go on in our world. A child who has been raped, his family murdered, him left to die of a lack of water in the desert must rather be dead than alive. These people are still blinded by the material. They do not believe in the everlasting glory of eternity, of which suffering is necessary, and that is fine. However, we must figure out how to convey to these people why this life is still better than no life at all."

"The default state of things is to not exist in the first place. Without the kickstart of the creator, everything could not have happened. Our souls reside in this blackness, until we burst forth in life within our mother's stomach. Suppose that suffering child were to look up at the sky and see the glorious blue powdered with the occasional wisp of cloud. For a second, not even a full one, he is able to enjoy the wonderfulness of this blessed earth created for us. That second, is worth far more than any blackness. That second, therefore, can outweigh the worst tortures of the world. A moment of happiness is all that is required to understand how much we take life for granted. Each time we draw breath is one we should revel in. The beauty in a single moment outweighs all the evils of man."

"One must love in order to reach this conclusion. Love is required to see the greatness in banality. Love is acceptance, and then revelation in the opportunity to do so. Love is the most important of the three for this reason. Love allows one to overcome the sufferings of the world, if only for an instant."

The crowd around Tazid, which had grew substantially as he gave his speech, stood up from their silence and cheered. The sun illuminated the holy man in a justified ring of heavenliness. He was still a man; that much was not in doubt. But now he was a man who steeled the hearts of many. Allowing them to face with bright eyes and smiles the death that was to come.

Arom stood up and asked the men (the bystanders and listeners to Tazid's sermon had departed to their various important chores at this point) whether he should fetch some fresh water. "We were going to today, before we got caught up in this mess."

Tazid had a moment of hesitation before responding, "You may die. In fact, its far more likely than not that will be the result."

"I understand. I wish to taste the sweet water of the earth our Lord has given us before I go. It is selfish, I'm aware. This is why I am asking the group. May I be allowed to revel in what I consider to be the one of the greatest gifts of God?"

The group collectively nodded. Who were they to deny this man his last drink? Arom went to his tent to don his armor.

Inside, Arom opened the holy book to the same passage Tazid had mentioned earlier. The Prophet had cited this line on more than one equation. Reading it gave Arom the strength to fulfill his final wish. He went on his knees and began to pray.

Thank you for this life Lord. I am sorry to lose what you have given me. Thank you for the time with my wife and children you gave me. I look forward to meeting them in heaven. Please keep them safe and tell them to wait only a little longer. I will be there with them soon. Amen.

Arom stood up smiling. It was time. He left his tent, said one final goodbye to the circle of men and friends, then walked to the edge of camp.

The army circled the camp in rectangular groups of a few hundred. The sandy hills rose to the lip of the valley, upon which the enemy stood. They had pitched a camp, only a few stood watch. They knew the camp in the valley wouldn't dare attack. They'd be massacred instantly. The archers on the ring of the valley lounged, not bothering to watch Tazid's group.

Arom asked himself whether he should run on crawl. Crawling would guarantee his safety to the water, but he would die like a snake. Slithering on the ground like a reptile with no backbone was not a proper way for a man to die. Arom readied himself. He drew in a deep breath to shout, "COME AND GET ME BASTARDS!"

A few of the archers on the hill slowly raised their heads. They had a look of surprise rather than annoyance. One little bug was not entertainment for them. The archers didn't know what he was doing. The limber man had no weapon on him. Was he suicidal? Some drew their bows as Arom ran toward the small creek that fell down one of the sandy ridges into a small, dirty pond.

Arrows began to fly at him. First it was only two, which he saw and dodged easily. Their high arc was easy to judge. The sand underneath Arom's bare feet was lose, yet he flew like a banshee. He had grown up in the sand, he knew how to run without getting caught. Each step brought Arom slightly closer to his goal. Gradually, more arrows flew at him. Arom had to make large zigzags in order to avoid them. His movement became more and more erratic.

Arom was only forty steps away from the pond when the first arrow struck him in the shoulder. That was fine, he didn't need his shoulder to run. He left the arrow in, it would be more incapacitating should he removed the barbed tip.

Twenty-seven steps and the next arrow hit him in the right arm. Again, he had no need for this body part. He could survive.

Twelve steps and a third hit him in the left shin. This one pierced all the way through, bringing Arom to his knees for a second. He stood up to keep moving. He was almost to the water. It wouldn't be long before he made it.

3 more steps, another arrow struck him in the same leg, rendering it completely unusable. Arom hobbled forward, falling face first to avoid several more tips raining down from the sky. He was at the water. Dunking his head under the surface, he took a huge gulp. He came up smiling.

Arrows showered his now still body. Giving him a porcupine look. The archers on the hill didn't bother going down to loot him. They would get their time eventually. They went casually back to their midday snoozing.

Arom closed his eyes and smiled. The thousand points of pain in his body didn't worry him. He could faintly hear in the distance the cheering of his peers. He wished they too would find their goal before the end came. Arom struggled to take in a final breath of God's air; his left lung struggled to hold it in. He shouted with as much force as he had before, "PRAISE BE TO GOD." Blackness overcame him. Arom was no more.

Tazid and the group had no tears in their eyes. Why would they cry when their friend had done what he desired? He had taken in the water of the divine, what could be better than that? The beauty in the ugliness and disgusting taste of the filthy mud ridden pond water was the cleanest taste Arom ever had.

Tazid turned back to his group, who were now joined by the rest of the camp on the western edge. He was going to give some more words of encouragement to the people, whose nerves were almost certainly shot. Then, one of the women pointed at the hill above where Arom died. "Look! What are they doing?"

Tazid gazed upon the sandy hill, squinting his eyes against the harsh sunlight. Down from the top rode the same band that had approach earlier with a promise of peace after surrender. The ugly man was again in the lead, smiling his disgusting grin. One of the men in the back carried a large wooden T.

They must really hate us if they're willing to use wood. Tazid stared at them, refusing to look away. Reaching the bottom of the hill, they lowered the cross onto the ground. Some of the men dug a hole in the sand, to make sure it wouldn't be knocked over. The thing was twice as tall as a man. Aroms body was turned over, the arrows pulled out with force. Blood oozed from the corpse slowly, covering Arom's clothing in a dark red. He was placed on the cross; his hands and feet nailed together with a crude hammer that looked more like a cudgel. The group raised the cross, displaying Arom's body for all to see.

The ugly man looked dissatisfied. He said something to the mercenary beside him. The man drew his scimitar as the leader shouted, "RESIST AND THIS WILL BE YOUR FATE, MEN." The sword wielder cut off Arom's head.

The cut was clean. The head fell straight onto the ground. The soldier picked it up by the mangled brown hair, now soaked wet with blood and the dirty water Arom had gleefully ran towards. The tongue was pulled out, and sliced off. One of the eyes was poked out with a few fingers. Then, the head was punted towards Tazid. Some teeth came flying out while the head travelled ungracefully in the air. The headless corpse stood woefully in front of them all, signaling the death of the camp. Arom's head lay in front of them, showing how twisted death would manifest.

Tazid bent over to say a prayer over Arom's head. He dug a small hole in the ground to bury it. When he finished, the bastard and his group were still there waiting patiently. The rest of the army on the hill had perked up at this point. Something entertaining was going on. One of the riders opened up a bottle to throw on Arom's body. Taking out a small device, he began striking sparks into the body. After five unholy minutes, the corpse went up in flames. The leader smiled again, and rode off, leaving the smell of Arom's burnt flesh to fill the air with its putrid stink.

The men sat around in a circle again. Tazid asked, "Does anyone have a wish they want to bring to fruition?" All of them shook their head. Unlike Arom, their families were all alive; most of them were in the camp. If they were to die, they would do so fighting.

The rest of the day was spent in merriness. The men got as drunk as they could without becoming so intoxicated they wouldn't be able to fight when the sun set. The women danced and sang songs. The children ran about gleefully. This was not a group that wanted to fight. It especially wasn't a group that wanted to survive. It was a collection of people who wanted to live. The ugly bastard who called down to them be damned.

The sun was about an hour from setting when all had finally settled down. Tazid gathered the camp in what would be their battle lines. They formed a circle around him. The innermost lining had the children. The second, the women. And defending them all, the men of all ages ringed the outside. Not a single person tried to escape. They were happy dying where they were, no matter how painful it would be. Tazid had them face him, and he gave his final sermon.

"What is there to say? I could guarantee you the eternal afterlife that is to come, but that would not do away with the pain you will face. The life after will be grand, you will bask in the infinitude of greatness that is God. This you already know and believe wholeheartedly. If it wasn't true, well, you wouldn't be here."

"I am grateful to have friends such as yourself. No. I am grateful people such as yourself graced me with your presence. The ability to stand firm against the onslaught is not one many people have. You all chose this, knowing the inevitable outcome. That is the true spirit of the human. To fight against the inevitable until the dying breath. To fight until the light fades away."

Sarai raised her eyebrows. "Rage until the dying of the light? That's a little plagiaristic my brown skinned friend, don't you think?"

"Shut up, racist." Said Pulp. He was oddly focused on the story. "Please continue. What happens next?"

"The chance of survival here is zero. Is that any different than the entirety of our existence? Not a single person will live forever. We do not have that capability. So why not embrace death fully, knowing the Lord is with us every step of the way? Many are not convinced of this idea. Many will fight against death in vanity, choosing the pleasure of the ground than the life eternal above. They have fallen into the mud to pick out a shiny rock. I hope our God forgives them for their transgressions."

"Does that make us good people? Not unless we are willing to say those engaged in sins are evil. That is perhaps the biggest crime of them all. Men cannot be evil or good. Men are just that, men—for when we assign the category of evil to another we have the imperative to destroy their lives, or, if they be good, to put them in the highest position of power. Only good people should be allowed to live, the evil ones should be killed. Thankfully, the Lord has not given us this. To have to discern who is evil from good would be an impossible task, ending in nothing but bloodshed. Seeing our incompetence in the calculation of right and wrong, the Lord has made all humans gray."

"Determining the value of the human, having been removed from us, can in no manner be the correct way to conduct ourselves in the world. What then, have we left to judge? Action."

"Those on the hill will say our actions our evil, therefore we too. The fallacy in their words is that humans cannot be evil. On this topic I have already spoken. More importantly, we move to the notion of collective guilt. The idea that one man is responsible for another is so blatantly prideful. It places one in the place of God. To think you have enough power to control others is to equivocate yourself to the divine who rules over all of us. We must not do this."

"Action has only to do with the individual. We are responsible for what each of us does individually. The actions we take are good and bad, they must be judged on that basis alone. When the end comes, God will tally these actions, as only he can determine the final weight. For us, we must take the actions as individual actions, and respond only with what is good—for to do a bad action is inherently a sin. To do a good action is to be righteous."

"The nonbelievers will come to us and ask, 'What makes an action righteous? You have no way of making that determination without committing the sin of pride.' Wrong. We have our determinate for us in the interpretation of the divine. There are a set number of ways in which we can interpret what the Lord has given to us. When he asks us to pray a certain way, he is by no means saying the moon is in fact a goddess of the hunt. Those two things cannot be related. We must begin by eliminating all possible wrongs, which will leave us with still myriad rights. From there, we take the right interpretations and see which ones are consistent with the rest of the teaching of God. The codification of consistency after elimination of all wrongness gives us the true doctrine. Again, the disbelievers will ask, 'How can you ever hope to achieve a momentous task? Once more, you are being prideful.' However, I have never claimed that I may be the one who determines the correct answer. All I can do is provide what I think is right, adding to the continual corpus of all human knowledge. Surely by compiling all that is known, eventually, we will come to the answer."

"Alas, we can no longer participate in this. I guarantee our story will be twisted and distorted. It will be used maliciously to describe how the unbelievers are horrid pigs that deserve slaughter. We will die without much consolation in this world (of which I have already addressed is not of the utmost importance)."

"But, I believe our story will be told. I believe there are people who will discover our tale for what it is. I believe beyond the odds that our tale will be told as it should. We must take solace in this. We must pray and ask that we become an example for the future generations. God willing, this must come to pass."

"We go happily to our deaths. I thank you for your devotion. I will die by your side, and see you on the other."

The crowd had eyes filled with tears, smiles as wide as rainbows, and cheers as loud as a thousand lions' roar. The sun sat in the background, and the slaughter began.

It was over much quicker than the enemy had hoped. While the lives were taken brutally, they were not carried out in the systematic way he had desired. The blasphemer, Tazid, was lost in the midst. No one found his body. The people were treated fairly. The women were barely raped. The children killed quickly. The men died valiantly. The fighting was over.

The army rode into the hot desert sun. The camels loped forward lethargically. They had begun to run out of water. In the distance, a low stone building came over the horizon. It was made of a blackish gray rock, with no adornments. Not far away, a small oasis came out of the sand. The water looked pure, so the army decided to rest there for the night.

Ank, the man tasked with carrying Tazid's head walked up to the fat leader under his open 1anopy. "Sir, there is a request from the monk inside."

Bart, the obese tyrant, looked up from the feast spread before him. He was wearing a beautiful set of robes, stained by the grease of animals. Two large breasted women sat on his lap, smiling and giggling. Their revealing garb disgusted Ank. It wasn't right the way he engaged in that horrific gluttony. Ank pushed it to the back of his mind.

Bart continued chewing, speaking with a full mouth, "What does he want?"

"He wants the pagan leader's head to bless."

Bart continued chewing. "Good, give it to him. If a man of that faith wishes to bless Tazid's headm they can. It will only serve to show how evil he truly was. Have the riders who looted come and pick it up."

"Yes, my lord." Ank left the tent to grab Tazid's head.

He walked through the camp, disappointed at what he saw. Bart wasn't the only one who engaged in those heathen activities. All throughout the camp he saw men and women drunkenly dancing. He heard screams from one tent as a naked woman burst out crying. The drunkard came after her, garbling filthy comments. Ank ignored it all.

He reached his tent, to thankfully find it had been left untouched. He kept his on the outskirts of the camp, where the few actual religious devotees lived. They stayed far away from the rowdiness, wanting to actually serve their lord. Their reason for coming wasn't one to fight, but one to spread to correct doctrine of the Lord. If they had to share company with pagans, so be it.

Ank got the sack in which the head was carried, a carefully wrapped woolen one. Upon reaching to the stone building he was greeted by the small old man he had met earlier. He had found the man's faith astounding, wanting to learn about it rather than kill him. While he disagreed with some of the man's tenants, the monk was a holy person. Ank knew that somehow.

"Here you are. Although, you know how many will perceive this."

The monk bowed his head in thanks. The bottom of his brown robes floated slightly off the ground, making the monk seem as though he levitated. "I'm aware. My Lord would be angry with me if I did not give a man of such conviction some holy rites, even if they aren't exactly his."

Ank nodded. "May I watch for a while? It would be good if someone of the faith were here to make sure you don't do anything vile."

Laughing good heartedly, the monk replied, "Vile? Do you presume me to be like those that lead your contingent?"

Ank's cheeks got red at the honesty more so than anger. "And what do you mean by that?"

"I think you know child. I'm not here to draw your ire. Come inside, I'll show you what I the Lord has commanded me to do." With that, the monk turned to the oak door (a wood rare as gold in the region).

The inside of the small temple was astounding only to those who entertain the idea of beauty within simplicity. There were three windows in all. Two clear glassed ones on the sides of the main room, one stain glass behind an altar. That alone was amazing. Glass was not meant for the poor. It took expensive blowers to make.

The altar was simple. It had two stone steps leading up to it. Stone benches carved out of the rock the room rose out of the ground to form several rows. Behind the altar was a cross. It was a simple, wood cross devoid of any figure. The stain glass behind it depicted a sun and two more crosses on either side. The one was slightly more illuminated than the other. The rest of the room was bare. There was no art, to tapestries, no rugs, no finery, no gold, nothing. It was vastly different than the places Ank had come to know as holy.

"I thought you worshipped the dead man, where is he?" Ank asked, genuinely curious. His previous apprehension about being caught in niceties with the monk was abandoned. There was something disarming about the man. Ank had no need to fear.

"Not quite, although those who lay claim to the head of our faith will tell you otherwise. We don't worship him, we walk hand in hand with him. His sacrifice, to take on all the sins of man, is not something out of the realm for you or I. He made the choice to give his body and blood for those he loved. Why can't you or I do that?"

Ank just shook his head. "We don't share the same God. You may walk with yours. To me, that's blasphemous. We serve our Lord."

"Why can't you do both? Do you serve your friends when you do good in their name? When you pledge to take care of a dying comrade's family, knowing the burden it will cause is great, are you not making the same sacrifice?"

"That's a commandment by God. He is not the same as us. I do not believe God can die, as yours did."

"God cannot die?"

"No." Ank said confidently.

"What happens when his name is no longer uttered?"

"That does not negate his existence."

"He no longer exists within the minds of men."

"That does not mean he exists outside the world of man."

"What proof do you have?"

"What proof do you have of your God?"

"I don't need proof. That's why there is no man on the wall. I may be wrong. The Lord may not have given his life, but I can. I can do good for my friends, and if need be, die in their name. I see no greater good than taking on the sins of others for the good of the world. If we all did so, the world would be a better place."

"The evil people would never consent."

"There are evil people? Says who?"

"Says God. Many of the disbelievers are evil, and should be purged to bring about utopia.”

“This isn’t utopia already?”

“How can you say such a thing? You see the death around us? You see the disease? The rape? The torture? The children who draw breath for one month before being brutally slaughtered? How can you even come close to calling this world perfect?”

The monk smiled. “The kingdom of God is all around us, we just can’t see it.”

“You are strange.” Ank replied.

The monk nodded. He moved toward the altar. Kneeling before it, he whispered a quiet prayer to the God he claimed could die.

The drawstrings of the bag came undone by the monk’s old hands. Inside was the head of Tazid. The dried blood around the neck hadn’t been cleaned up. His eyes were open, the pupils were disintegrating into goo. Miraculously, no flies or bugs had gotten inside the bag. The hair was matted with sweat. Its black curls tangled like a mangy dog. The monk put the head down on the stone block of the altar, under the cross. He sat there, praying.

Ank stood there for a half hour before interrupting. “Is that all you plan to do?”

The monk nodded without breaking his concentration.

Ank decided to stay watch. He was charge of the head and had nothing better to do. The camp didn’t particularly need him for anything other than this task. Even then, he had only been chosen by luck of the draw.

The young warrior took a seat in the back of the room. He began his own contemplations. Night came a few hours later. Ank left temporarily for dinner. He came back with an extra bowl of stew for the monk. The man still knelt in front of Tazid’s head. Ank wondered what could have possibly been so great about the blasphemer.

“Monk, I’ve brought you dinner.” This time, the holy man stopped his prayer. He retrieved the bowl, said a thanks, and ate.

“Why do you care for him so much?” Ank inquired. Over the several hours of thought, he drew no conclusions about why a lone man of another faith would value the dead leader of a faulty group.

Waiting until his mouth was empty, the monk gave the speech that would change the course of Ank’s, and all who shared his faith, forever.

“He isn’t different than you or I. Tazid was just a man. That’s why I value him. He is not his deeds, those are apart from him. You look at the two as the same. The man is that which he does. My God does not teach that. We are who we are, nothing else. The things we do have no bearing on our worth."

"Tazid's actions are what I admire. They were great deeds. This head symbolizes them. He was kind in a world where the down and out are rejected. His example is one that is echoed through the ages as impressive, yet so few undertake the task of following in the archetypal footsteps. Tazid tried to free an entire people with no more than a few fighting men. He knew the outcome. He went anyways. His followers were so impressed they stayed with him until their horrific dying breath."

"He lived like his life was not his own. The life didn't belong to a state or some worldly entity, but to God. Within that framework he acted according to divine command. There is no other way to live."

The two stayed in prayer over the head of Tazid for two more days. In the end, after three passed, Tazid retrieved the head. He managed to lose it halfway through the journey in a simple grave, marked by an olive tree. Ank spent the rest of his life learning the deeds of Tazid. He spread this knowledge to everyone he could before being martyred on the same cross as the monk's dead God.

Interlude 10

Kant: Called it.

Chris: That's rather hopeful.

Ali: Don't sacrifice yourself for some vain god. You are the vain god. Satisfy yourself.

Chris: That's not what I meant.

Triangle: Chris is right. Who wouldn't want that end?

Doc: Triangle, if I have to patch you up again I'll give you an end myself. Stop your martyrdom.

Triangle: No.

Divo: Now that's poetic.

Cortez: I enjoyed that story. Mercenaries are bad, but zealots are worse.

Chris: Mercenaries aren't zealots for money?

Diog: No, that's lawyers.

Doc: You're a lawyer.

Diog: Yup.

Doc: You statists are horrible.

Kant: Kind of hard to make a categorical claim like such.

Dmitri: Holy shit.

Sumac: Is Dmitri or Kant next?

Dmitri: Not I.

Kant: This one is for the crazies in here. Perhaps you'll see some of yourself in our protagonist.

The Honest World

"People are divided as good and evil. The line between such is easily delineated when we observe the objective rules of the universe. Thus, it is so we shall seek to eliminate all possible evil by removing those who commit it. While theorists in the past have."

The professor droned on while Jordan paid no attention in the back row. This type of moral education was just the repeating of the same lesson they had learned for decades. If you go against the rules, you die. Pretty simple. And the number one rule?

"What would that be Jordan?"

"To always tell the truth in every situation."

"And is that any different form Kantian ethics?"

"In regards to the truth? No. There is no excuse for telling a lie, no matter what the circumstance." That, however, had been a lie Jordan repeated back to his teachers for years. The issue with lying, as had been deduced many years ago, is that it caused a twisting of reality. In the past, this had been a huge problem for societies. People would espouse perceived truth rather than truth itself. This allowed the most cunning of all to rise to the top, slowing societal progress. Wars were fought over things a proper grasp on morality could have solved. It is only because people lied, there was war.

After the near destruction of the planet, a race from above had stepped in. No one actually remembers this time, as it is left mysteriously blank in all but a few texts. The rest of world history still existed, but the rift provided one of the only sources of debate still in existence. What happened?

No one knew, nor would anyone ever know. But what was certain is that by speaking an untruth, anyone over the age of 26 would immediately disappear. The leeway of 26 years was thought to be because of the age at which a brain achieves maturity. However, a problem was presented to the higher race (some people thought the higher race possessed the ultimate moral knowledge, and hence, this wasn't actually a problem). What do you do with the intellectually incompetent? Can you blame a moron for telling a lie? Or what about mental illness? The question of a "rational actor" that philosophers so love to discuss was brought to the forefront of the moral landscape.

The answer was blunt. When a woman, or anyone else found out an infant would be born with a defect, the thing would not exist in the morning. There wasn't any sign of trauma, surgery, or anything else for the imagination. In much the same was as people, these children just up and disappeared.

People didn't know the reasons why the higher race made its choices, but many tried deducing the reasoning from the conclusion. On the extreme end of things (what was becoming an all too common mindset) there were those who thought of disabilities as corruption of man. Any negative adaptation, as judged by the higher race, was wrong. For whatever reason, the existence of any wrongness must be eliminated. This mindset had taken root rather quickly, it made one question the goodness in man's heart, something eerily reminiscent of WWIII.

What had brought the third world war was a belief there were good and bad people. And what is the charge of the good? To destroy all bad. It was a simple formula that takes hold whenever one is certain of good and wrong in the world. Fortunately, this mindset was mitigated by the benevolence of the higher race. By having a moral arbiter remove all imperfections, men could consider one another good.

Another group of people saw the higher race as wicked puppet masters playing God. Surprisingly, they weren't eliminated when they spoke openly about their hatred. In fact, many people who committed the worst acts of all were spared. Their mortal body remained to be punished by the society around them.

The rules on what constituted truth were still being discovered, and hence big problems in the world of law were manifested. First, the issue of guilt. If one believed another to be guilty, it was often not enough. Many judges and jurors were zapped from the earth because they declared guilt despite their doubt. More people than ever were set free as they could not be convicted. Secondly, sentencing became complicated. One could no longer equate the pain caused by the accused to the pain the state would inflict. This required a value schema too complex and nonsensical that even more judges were eviscerated. Societies all around the globe figured out fast the only two possible solutions. Rehabilitation was put into practice more and could be used even when one was unsure of guilt. For crimes such as rape, murder, pedophilia, and the like, Hammurabi's Code was reinstituted. Castration for sexual predators, death for the murderer, and burning for the arsonist. Before the higher race entered into the world, ethical arguments against this were valid. However, with absolute certainty that death comes with untruth, one could be certain that all else was in some way truthful. No judge who had sentenced a pedophile to castration had been removed.

A final group of people chose to go into hiding. They stayed in the fringes of hospitable landscapes, praying to their strange gods. Jordan actually came from a town close by to one of these villages. When he was a kid, the village youth would frequently visit the strangers for fun, learning the bizarre ways of the people. The kids were always told never to trust the words of the savages, because they could lie. Jordan liked listening to their stories. He never once heard an outlander tell a lie. He heard stories upon stories of great tales of adventures, heroes, monsters, demons, damsels, and all the like. By the time he left for school, Jordan had an immense repertoire of knowledge codified in stories.

The knowledge tended to manifest itself in the life of Jordan. He got up at an early hour, meditated, did his language skills, worked out, all before seven. He was kind to others, although not entirely sure why. He made sure to save money whenever he got any. (With the new world, this was not unique to Jordan. Money had become one of the only ways of telling status, and so many people began to save more and more. Decentralized currency, gold, and even fiat saw a huge boost in investment from non-liquidated capital to pure financial investments.)

Jordan called his family twice a week. Back home, his parents were physicians. His dad, Chuck, took care of minor injuries and long-term illness. He was well loved among the community. Jordan's mom, Amelia, was an emergency physician. She never gained much popularity because her primary job was yelling at drunks to hold still on the table. Jordan took special care when talking to his family. His brother was far too good at everything, so Jordan made sure to cautiously praise and simultaneously point out flaws. Jordan's brother deeply looked up to him. His sister had faced serious trouble in her life. She had a series of unfortunate events occur in her youth, leading to a mental cascade. That was another quirk of the truth telling system, the mentally ill got a pass. Not that she would have been killed, but it was a constant note of assurance that needed to be given to Bug. She hated that name, but Jordan called her it anyways.

One couldn't help but conclude Jordan was a good person. In nearly all realms he excelled. Jordan, however, failed in what mattered most at school: social skills. Jordan had friends, but they were few and far between. Of the several in his hometown, he wanted to marry one. She was the perfect match for Jordan (in his mind, at least). His favorite movie when younger was an old film his dad made the whole family watch on many occasions. The main character, a farm boy, would profess his love by responding to the farmer's daughter, "as you wish." Even Jordan knew this was too cheesy to do in real life. Instead, Jordan took to driving her around and paying for all her meals. He indulged her sometimes horrible taste in music in the car rides up and down the endless roads. All of it was done out of love. Jordan's other closest friend went to a less well-off school nearby. He was probably smarter than Jordan, and deserved to be where Jordan was. He excelled at making friends. He couldn't walk into a room without lighting up the whole place. Given his tragic past, it was a wonder he managed such a feat. Jordan looked up to him and aspired to be as good as he was.

Nowadays, things were vastly different. Jordan sat in a cold basement room typing, reading, and wasting time more than anything else. He had begun to despise himself. His routine was monotonous, and he had no one to whom he could talk. The world was slowly getting darker, and he knew it.

Jordan had joined a better than average university in one of the country's central hubs. The constant busyness of people betrayed how little they accomplished. Students and local shopkeeps seemed to do the most work. Students of the university, and others nearby, were kept under constant surveillance at the school. Cameras spread like fleas in everywhere except the bathroom stalls. The purported goal of the setup was to aggregate the nature of truth itself.

It was conceived not long after many of the university's utopians disappeared. Deriving value from facts without an interpretative framework was fundamentally wrong according to the higher race. Religious professors also disappeared rather quickly. That one was more difficult to handle.

Thoughts like these permeated Jordan's head when he sat mentally alone at the desk. Boredom so strong took a hold of him he was forced to think of ridiculous things. Why can't I just accept the way things are? His parents told him that when their grandparents were alive, that's what people were told to do. They were supposed to love themselves for who they were. The higher race changed that as well. Those who told others they are fine just the way they are, were entirely gone. Most of the disappeared came to be so via this route. The denial the ideal future is the present, was utterly ridiculous.

Class ended and Jordan stepped on the bus to go to work. Another series of mind numbing hours was to occur. Jordan had tried to write essays in his mind, but he saw pictures instead of words. The pictures were rarely controllable, despite their high resolution. The bus stopped, Jordan hopped off, and entered the grey building.

The air was slightly frosted. Looking to the sky, it was as though a dome covered the Earth. The blanket of snow hiding in the heavens was soon to smother the ground. The pure crystals of water would be greeted with concrete and the collective moral destitute of a society.

The cubicle was simple and white. Small walls on three sides hid workers from each other. Jordan hated it. He thought he would be a man's man like his father, but he needed people. It took Jordan a long time to figure out the meaning of his need. He didn't want constant conversation, unless about ideas. He didn't want a group. Most of all, he didn't want to be a replaceable cog in a group. That was scariest of all. The boss probably picked up on Jordan's dislike of the environment.

All of a sudden, while lost deep in thought, Jordan missed the Chief of

Staff staring at him. "What the hell are you doing?"

"Thinking."

"Get back to work." The portly man had an air of arrogance. His sweaty, fat face sought power alone. Jordan though he should start with his diet, a view not shared by the Pig. Jordan knew his name but outright refused to call him anything other than "boss". The savages had taught him names should be descriptive. Jordan had taken kindly to the idea, proceeding to give mental names to everyone he encountered. Occasionally he would tell the person, usually not to a good result.

Again, Jordan's mind trailed off. There wasn't actually any work to do. It's possible that the city creates work for itself to complete, never getting anything done. The perpetual loop of non-responsibilities being completed by non-caring individuals was utterly repulsive to Jordan. He hated how no one took the initiative. Instead, blame would be placed upon others. Another quirk of the higher race's system was that those who took responsibility for the things outside their control did not disappear. Jordan took this approach begrudgingly.

The day passed by slowly. The pace of the ticking clock slowed with each passing minute. Calls came infrequently, emails were sparse, and the place had nothing to do.

Around three in the afternoon, Jordan was called into his boss's office. Jordan's direct boss, wasn't there. Rather, his boss's boss sat in his boss's chair.

"Do you know why I called you in here today?"

"I think you're gonna let me go."

"Why?"

Jordan paused for a second. He was still young enough to give him a chance at lying. Unlike many of the others, he had done so a fair amount. Having everyone assume you're telling the truth is a useful tool.

"You don't like me. You don't have any real reason to fire me, as I have given you none. But, you don't like me and want to show how powerful you are." Jordan also took advantage of the greatest flaw in the system; If you confront someone with something that encompasses the whole truth, they can't deny it. For example, if Jordan had just shook his head and said no, the boss could have said, "It's because of your age boy. We don't hire people as young as you around here." Which would have been partially true. But, it didn't tell the whole truth. What Jordan had said was entirely true, and the boss knew it. He angrily looked Jordan in the eyes, "Get the fuck out of this office."

Jordan took the comment in stride and replied coolly, "Only if you get the fuck out of the female interns." Jordan had no idea whether this was true. It would certainly piss the boss off, and that's all that mattered. The boss guided him out of the door and grumbled, "You have ten minutes before I call the police." The wooden door slammed hard against Jordan's back. Some others in the office looked up only briefly. The boss did these things all the time.

Jordan hid his anger and sadness behind a veneer or stoicism. On the outside, he looked as he always did, with a resting face that displayed a mild and mute anger. It was enough to satisfy the inner rage. Jordan grabbed his things as casually as possible and put them in his bag. He put his coat on, and turned to leave. Passing by the front lobby, he grabbed the entire jar of watermelon candies and marched out the doors.

The cold air hit him like a truck. The office building was kept at a summer temperature. The outside kept it at freezing. Snot and tears froze almost immediately. One couldn't walk outside without a foot of layers on. Jordan waddled to the bus stop, huddling underneath the flimsy plastic roof over the bench. He sat beside a small elderly woman. She curled in an almost fetal position. Strange thoughts about mortality and the old lady's fetal look passed in Jordan's head. Maybe you should return her where she belongs. She looks like she wants to be there. Might as well say fuck the boss by leaving a body at the door. Jordan felt the knife he kept in his jacket pocket. It was big enough to take out the woman. A stab in the neck would be all it takes. What the hell are you thinking? What if the blizzard let up for a second and someone saw?

Jordan's worries didn't manifest. In defiance of his thoughts, the blizzard picked up. More white snow whipped around in the dark evening. Jordan sat on the knife's edge of a choice. He was saved by the faint lights and low rumble of a bus plodding along the icy road. The bus slowly pulled up to the stop and let out a few passengers. Jordan noticed the old lady hadn't gotten up from her position. He pushed her a little.

"What are you pushing me for you bastard?"

"The bus is here."

"And what makes you think I don't just want to stay and freeze?"

"Suit yourself." Jordan started up the steps. He showed the driver his pass and took a seat in the front row. No one else was on the bus, as was typical. Most people in the office would be there until dawn. The buses to and from the station would be empty until an hour before sunrise. Jordan had never taken the bus at this hour before. He found it quite peaceful.

He popped his headphones in and started the classical music. He had been listening to the stuff for a half decade now, and still hadn't taken the time to learn any of the songs. He could recognize them, but not the composer or title. When walking around, it felt as though a band was behind you, scoring your life. Jordan enjoyed that greatly. He could never focus anyways when there were lyrics. The incessant whining intrinsic in modern music's lyrics was incredibly annoying. The classical had arguably gotten worse as well, but at least it could pass as art. The wailing of the moderns lies in the same category as the sexual moaning of a dying cat.

The old lady walked slowly onto the bus. The cold had sunk into her bones. Jordan wondered whether it was the day's cold, or a lifetime that caused her to look so shriveled and stiff. She took a seat several behind Jordan. He heard her hard breathing faintly, and so turned up his music.

The bus started up, the driver taking another sip of sludge from his thermos. "Next stop, Grenwood." Jordan had about an hour before he got home. He wiped off some condensation off the window. The outside world hid everything. The occasional lights of passing cars would reveal the deep snow along the side of the road. The well salted highways started gathering more and more ice. The stars, which were normally so bright, couldn't pierce the blizzard. The driver wisely turned off the high beams.

Doing so brought Jordan back to his childhood. His father taught him to drive during a storm similar to this. He drove him up to the elementary school with its big parking lot. With his kind, gruff voice, Dad had told him to floor it.

"What? Why? It's icy."

"I know. How else are you gonna learn?"

Jordan sure as hell hoped the bus driver had a similar father. That past morning skidding across the icy asphalt taught Jordan how to control the vehicle and how to stay calm in terrifying situations.

The bus pulled up to another stop. Jordan barely registered it. His mind was racing through thoughts tempered by the music. It was the last time he'd ever have to make the long journey to the opposite side of the city.

A man wearing a black hoodie, black pants, black backpack got on the bus. He sat directly adjacent to Jordan, never looking up. He too slipped on some headphones. Jordan was half surprised he didn't try to rob the three other people on the bus. Maybe there just weren't enough victims and he gave up upon seeing their sorry state. The old lady was half dead, the bus driver was on the come down from some stimulant, and Jordan was ready to release his anger in a violent rage. It wasn't the best score for the criminal.

Jordan turned up his headphones yet again and passed out.

He awoke with some screaming he didn't recognize. The language was harsh. Each syllable cut the eardrums with a gravelly fury. Jordan got the message. He took out his headphones and lay on the ground with his hands covering his neck. Well, it's an exciting last day.

The man who looked like a criminal lay behind Jordan. The terrorist was done investigating his captives. The terrorist had no desire to steal; he wanted to kill. As he raised the Kalashnikov, the criminal shot him with a gun he quickly drew from his pants.

Blood erupted from the man's chest. The terrorist's snowy white clothing became matted with crimson, his long. His scraggly beard became dyed with the man's own life. Jordan stood up, wiping the dirt from his clothes. "You really ought to clean your bus, the ground is absolutely filthy."

The bus driver, who had somehow survived, calmly replied, "Why would I clean filth for filth?"

"Are you calling me filth?"

"No. Just humanity."

The world of crime had a significant change since the higher race came. Only sociopathic murderers could get away with something anymore. The threat, "If you don't give me the money, I'll kill you" was so often an empty one before. Petty criminals had a huge chunk taken out of the population. After about a year, the higher ups in crime syndicates realized they needed to employ those who stuck to their word. In the business of death, that was sociopaths.

The number of veterans on the streets rapidly disappeared. The country solved one problem, while another one was created. The veterans were retrained, put on psychotropics, and sent to run wild. The mind was in a state of haziness on the drugs, never fully remembering anything. Essentially, the criminal lords created supersoldiers by breaking a man down as much as possible, first with war and then with drugs. The PTSD veterans were now aim and kill machines, like the one who had tried to take over the bus.

It would be wrong to limit this phenomenon to the criminal elements of society. Often the government would retrain the same veterans for similar purposes. The broken men could be used to infiltrate and execute plots all across the globe. Western countries managed to hide the worst of it all. The totalitarian ones created entirely new military systems. The newest soldiers would be sent to the front lines, in the worst possible conditions—just enough to plant the seed of uncertainty about reality itself. Then, they would send in the previously broken soldiers to clean up the mess. Wars were fought by the damned, the spoils won by the damners. At least there was one fewer heroin addict to throw on the pile.

Jordan got up and moved back several seats. The terrorist's body was going to lie there until the driver finished his shift. People missed seeing blood. The bleakness of the world set in on humanity more and more. It seemed as though people had reached an age when the chaos had subsided, leaving in its wake the ashes of human spirit. Mankind was given rules to follow, and from these rules a new order was to emerge. However, the current state of affairs did nothing more than kick the ashes in the air. Some willfully shoved it in their eyes and ears.

To Jordan, it seemed like the world had gotten worse since the higher race came. People no longer created. The artists put down their brushes. The musicians gave up their instruments. Authors renounced the pen. People were cowards. They had become so scared of the possibility of falsely manifesting the truth, they became scared of truth itself.

Jordan had sympathy for the creators. They had long since disavowed their practice. The greats were never liars, at least in their work. Monet, Da Vinci, Michelangelo, Dali, and the rest of the creators told the truth in their art. Individually, they may have made shite choices. It does not mean the art cancels those choices out. In those actions, the creators twisted reality. In their art, they described it as truthfully as possible.

That really is the difference between art and propaganda. But now all was neither. It was a reflection of an aesthetic's soul. Jordan used to like this idea. The notion of burning it all to the ground and to keep burning it until the very earth singed black, was a nice idea. In practice it fell. You run out of things to burn. You end up immolating yourself.

Jordan believed this to be the cause of society's soon to be collapse. The destruction of the lie created fear where it should have created courage. Man no longer went willingly into the dark. Every day was a continual rehashing of the same lessons, the same work, the same, the same, the same, the same, the same. Fucking a, even the bus rides were relatively the same. The crazed bastards on psychotropics were common. Everyone carried a piece. Funny how in a world of normalcy the crazies were largely ignored. The higher race didn't achieve their goal; they didn't create a world of truth. They created a world of invertebrate cowards.

The bus pulled up to Jordan's stop. He calmly thanked the bus driver and stepped out into the brisk dark. Only a small station bench was illuminated by the dingy streetlight above it. Under the flickering, a small woman sat. She reminded Jordan of the older woman from before. The spirit of Raskolnikov fought for its control. Jordan turned around and walked in the opposite direction.

All about him were choices. All were truthful. All were valid. Does that mean all were good? The correlation between the good and the truth became…

Jordan thought these thoughts to distract himself. Deep in his own mind, Jordan stepped to a crossing. The universal red stopped him. On the other side of the road Jordan saw a biker pick up speed to cross. Her thin tires left the faintest tread on the grey snow. She and her bike were beautiful. The circling of the wheels was mesmerizing. The beauty of something so simple wasn't lost on Jordan.

The biker got halfway across the street before he was run over.

The truck could give two shits. From the void of the night, the black vehicle sent the biker flying into the air. The truck didn't stop.

Jordan ran over to the young woman. She looked about his age. Ragged breathing came from what looked to be a face. The mangled body of what once was a human being would invoke fear in the strongest of physicians. Her bones poked out. Her twisted legs twitched like a cricket. Jordan picked her up and carried her off the road. He sat down on the curb, holding the lady's head in his arms. She looked terrified.

"It will be alright, I promise. Close your eyes and focus." She responded by shutting her eyes. Jordan pulled out some watermelon candies. "Open your mouth." Jordan slowly unwrapped the red paper and place the candy on her tongue. "See? Life is sweet." She nodded. Jordan reached around his back under his overcoat.

"And what the hell are you doing there that night?"

"I was walking back to my apartment."

"You keep saying that and I still don't believe you."

"Suit yourself."

"Don't you want a lawyer kid?"

"No."

"Do you want an adult?"

"I am an adult."

"What about your family, what will they think when they find out you murdered a young woman?"

"I didn't murder her."

"Yes, I think you did. Many people think you did."

"Since when is truth determined by majority consensus?"

"Since when is a bullet hole in the head classified as anything but murder?"

Jordan stopped talking. This was getting nowhere. They had no evidence. After ending her painful life, Jordan called the police. Rashly, he forgot to pick up the shell. That's how they got him. The sirens (Jordan thought it funny how Sirens are creatures of death. Fitting that a cop should use them.) blared through the night. When the cops came, Jordan was asked to come in for questioning. Several hours later, he was still sitting in the interrogation room with two officers.

The one asking the questions was a short, fat, ugly man. He looked like one who hated life. He clearly didn't take care of his own. The doughy officer paced around the room while talking. Occasionally he would hit the table in anger.

The other officer sat nicely at the table. He smiled at Jordan, offering him a glass of water.

"No, thanks."

"Suit yourself." The spindly man made the pair look straight out of a comedy sketch. Frankly, Jordan found the whole situation extremely entertaining. The law had faced continual struggle when trying those from the age of 18 to 26. They could still lie, and had no obligation to tell the truth.

"Why was she so mangled?"

"She was biking. She crossed the street, and was hit by a truck."

"Why didn't you say something?"

Jordan didn't respond again. The question was a trap. The why of something in these legal matters ends up fucking the defendant in the long run. Never answer the question why. Jordan ran through all his legal classes and felt falsely confident in his own intellectual prowess.

"I want a lawyer."

"Well you can't have one right now." Should the fat man had left out the part, "right now" he would have vanished.

"Then I will not respond to any further questions."

The fat man started to say something but as interrupted by the spider. "I think we're done here. You're free to go."

Jordan nodded and pushed back the hard metal chair. He walked towards the door only to be slammed against the table by the fatty. "Did you kill that woman?"

Jordan didn't respond. The sweat dripping from the man got Jordan's face wet. The other cop took out his pistol and whipped the fat one.

"I'm sorry. I want truth, he wants to be right." The cop was genuinely apologetic.

"No worries."

At home, Jordan couldn't shower off the stench of the dead woman or the fat man. The aroma created was one of fear, disgust, and confusion. I did the right thing. I did the right thing. I did the right thing. Over and over again the words ran through Jordan's skull. They failed to assuage the slightest of fears.

The steam from the shower fogged the mirror. Jordan stepped out of the shower, his muscled body dripping. He grabbed a towel dried himself down. Jordan stood in front of the mirror, wiping away some of the condensation.

What stared back at him was inhuman. The high cheekbones and dark golden eyes were uncaring. The black beard added another layer of evil to the portrait.

"What have I done…"

"WHAT HAVE I DONE." Jordan raised his fist to pummel the glass. Whatever that was, was not supposed to be here. Jordan learned from past experience this wasn't a good idea. His fists still bore the scars of previous mirrors.

"Fuck."

Jordan threw on some grey sweatpants and went to the living room. The walls were plain. The room had a low brown table in front of a ratty couch. The couch faced a giant screen. Jordan and the screen shared many nights together. No one else would. The company they kept each other was beautiful. Electronics didn't care what you did. No matter who you were, you were nothing to the screen.

Jordan flicked on some nature documentary about spiders. The researcher held up a dark, hairy creature. "This ere, is one of the most venomous spiders in the world. And I'm gonna touch it." Another man entered the frame. He was of tanned skin. He wore a beige safari hat, brown gumboots, and some foreign outfit.

"There aren't many of these fellas left in the world. They only live ere in this sanctuary, and maybe out in the nearby jungle. They only hunt at night. There entire life is spent in the dark. This one here is a female, all the big ones are. The males are about the size of a pinhead; their only purpose is to procreate. The females do all the work."

"Must be a shit society if the women have to do all the heavy lifting." Jordan said out loud, laughing to himself. In a response, the universe gave Jordan a hard knock on the door.

"Who is it?" He shouted over the television.

"Jordan Eschew, please open the door." The pounding continued, only harder this time. Jordan got up lazily. He turned the brass handle slightly to be shoved down to the floor.

"Jordan, you are under arrest for the murder of Lily Lash." The bulky officer turned him around. "Put your hands behind your back." Jordan did as he was told.

"I didn't murder her."

"And if you were twenty-six, you would have disappeared. You fucking minors lie, lie, lie. We should lock you all in a cage."

The iron cell door creaked open, and Jordan was thrown against the wall. "Here's your food maggot."

Jordan rushed over to the food, licking up the last remains. A hard roll of bread, grey soup, a rotten apple, and juice didn't do much to assuage the pain throughout the Jordan's body. He had been beaten mercilessly by the guards. They really were convinced he killed the girl. This was the treatment murderers got, not someone who called the police.

Blood slowly pooled from a wound on Jordan's leg. He ripped off his left sock to tie it around. It wasn't much of a tourniquet, but it stopped the bleeding. The last few days were all blurs. After being arrested, Jordan was told he'd have to wait a week before a trial. A whole fucking week (Jordan didn't know back in the day waiting for the trial sometimes took years). He had slept six times, but that could mean anything. His brains had been scrambled to the point of near incomprehension. He couldn't hold a thought for more than a minute. The only thing that gave him comfort was the darkness of the cell. He could hide from everything there. The guards never beat him in his room; there he was safe.

Jordan's hallucinations came back the minute he was arrested. He felt long cuts on his wrists and neck, without anything there. The burning sensations overwhelmed him at night. The respite of the room was soon substituted with the torture of the Jordan's mind. His anxiety, being through the roof, took ahold of his person. Jordan wasn't Jordan. He was some sort of anxiety-ridden monster, ready to bite at the slightest provocation.

He had managed a fight during his only outside hour earlier in the day. Another inmate kept calling him murderer (how he knew about the situation was anyone's guess) and shouting obscenities from a bench. Jordan walked over and asked if something was the matter.

"You killed a fucking child."

"No, I didn't."

"You know you're an evil person?" The man disappeared form sight.

"Hey man, what the fuck did you do? Jimmy just disappeared!" One of Jimmy's friends walked toward Jordan.

"Did you make him tell a lie you cunt?"

"With my power to control the minds and mouths of others? Yes. You caught me. I'm a sorcerer."

"How the fuck did you not disappear?" The gentleman clearly had a poor understanding of the universal rules.

"Like I said, I'm a magician."

"Stop fucking with me."

"Or what? You'll beat me? I'm deeply terrified of an overly built man who hasn't done any cardio in the past decade."

The man raised his arm to swing, but Jordan ducked under it. The punch was hard, but slow. As long as Jordan kept his speed, he should be good. The bigger man followed with a knee to Jordan's head. Jordan spun away, getting behind Jimmy's friend. Jordan swept out the man's legs, and watch him fall hard to the ground.

"You good?"

"Like hell I am."

The guy drew out a shiv. Now things are getting interesting thought Jordan. His senses were overwhelmed with adrenaline. For the first time in a month he felt something other than despair.

The man got up and made a stab at Jordan. Jordan danced lightly backwards. His years of working out coupled with martial art training kicked in. He never made in far in any discipline, but compiled the basics of everything from judo to aikido.

Again, another stab with the disgusting looking knife. This time, Jordan grabbed the man's wrist. He used the momentum to flip the larger man over his head and again onto the ground. The shiv came loose from hands and Jordan kicked it away.

"Sir, are you fucking done? I just had to pull some Bruce Lee shit and do not appreciate being attacked."

"Who the fuck is Bruce Lee?"

"Your worst nightmare." Jordan kicked the guy in balls. He watched him writhe in pain as guards ran up behind him.

"That's it, no more outside time for you today."

Jordan ran through the memory in his head. It was so recent, it was all Jordan had to hold on to. Remembering the beatings would only serve to cause more pain. Try to forget everything and Jordan would lose himself.

In quiet contemplation, Jordan nursed his aches with meditation and massage. The water pouring from the sink did some to assuage his pain. He used his other sock as a towel to wipe the water from his face.

Jordan crawled over to the slightly raised bead on a metal frame. Laboriously, he pulled himself onto the cement the guards called a mattress.

Jordan saw a man enter through the door. He had a long black beard, and a tan complexion. Jordan sat straight up. He had no pain anywhere. When Jordan pinched himself, he felt nothing.

"I'm dreaming, aren't I?"

The man answered, "Does that make it any less real?"

Jordan shook his head. He tried looking at the figure some more, but whenever he focused too much his eyes were struck with a brilliant light. The man was bathed in it.

"Don't you think this is a little too on the spot for a Christophanoy?"

"Probably."

"Why?"

Christ sat down cross-legged on the floor. "Will you listen to me?"

"I don't think I stand much of a chance against the divine, do I?"

"I would never consider enacting violence on you, nor would God. May I ask, have you ever read Jonathon Livingston Seagull?"

"You know the answer, being timeless redemption and all. Yes, I have read that book in secret. It took me a long time to get, most places outright ban it."

"And what was the lesson of that book?"

"All men have the spirit of flight within them, it is only by looking at material is the spirit destroyed."

"Did you read the final chapter?"

"No, it was ripped out."

"The final chapter goes something like this: Jonathan becomes the king of the seagulls. His friends start to spread his word—only it grows more and more fantastical. Elements of Jonathan's life are removed, supplanted by glorious tales of miracles. Eventually, a myth about Jonathan's eyes begins to spread and people place their focus on this insignificant part of his life. A cult of Jonathan begins to worship him as a hero. And was Jonathan a hero? Yes. Was he the hero? No. That was the fundamental confusion is the same with the masses. I am no longer one to emulate, I have become one to worship. Nothing has ever been farther from the truth. Man is already fully God. He is not fully man.

"Your higher race was meant to guide you toward salvation, instead it led you into the arms of the stoics. No longer can one feel pure joy or suffering, instead you subsist on the greyness of life. Pure joy or suffering cannot be expressed rationally without one considering it "lying". What is rational about suffering? Biologically all are suffering at all times. Is that all there is to suffering? No. It is something too of the spirit, the unconscious mind. One cannot tell others of this deep and dark suffering without art, or an attempt to find the truth. By punishing those who seek the truth and reach a misguided answer, no one wants to be truthful anymore. Instead, it is a mere obligation to find truth. I'm sure you're wondering what happens to those who are whisked away for lying?"

Jordan nodded.

"They are placed in a room like this one. It is purely black; light does not exist in that place. When they are taken out of the room, they are blindfolded.

Never again are they allowed to see light. They are chained up to the ceiling and floor. Then, they are tortured. It usually takes a few days to find out what hurts them the most. Sometimes it is pulling nails. Sometimes it is extracting teeth with a knife. For others, it is flayed skin or the whip. Still more detest boiling water. The worst, is what they do to the face. Skin is peeled away again and again, never able to fully regrow. The nose is cut with a rusty blade. One eye is put out eventually. At some point, they take the tongue— but never the fingers or toes. Pulling nails is too much fun for them. They enjoy it. The prisoners all break. Their mind leaves this realm and makes its way to purgatory. There, they wait for someone to redeem their soul."

Jordan interrupted, "Isn't that your job?"

The room shook as Christ spoke. "No. I am not your redeemer. Why are you turning to the divine exterior rather than that which lies within yourself? Make yourself free."

"How do I do that?"

"Follow the Word of the Lord." The room went dark and Jordan shot straight up. Sweat poured down his face. He looked down at himself, realizing his wounds really were gone.

No way that could have happened.

The door creaked slightly open. No one came in. Jordan shuffled quietly to peer through the crack. No one was in the hall. The wailing of the other prisoners was the only sound. The corridor was lit by a fluorescent white light. Jordan pushed the door open and walked into the light. He reached the end of the cement hall to a chain-link gate. What the hell am I supposed to do now? Jordan looked around until he saw the maintenance closet.

He tried to open the door, only to realize it was locked. Jordan kicked the hinges. The sound wouldn't be heard by the guards over the wailing of other inmates. The door budged slightly. He kicked again, and again, and again. The door groaned backwards, hanging lose from the frame. Inside the closet were the mop bucket, a mop, and an assortment of other small things. Jordan grabbed the mop, running to the chain-link. The mop handle was metal; it broke the door easily. (Why was the mop handle metal? So inmates couldn't make shanks out of splinters.)

Jordan ducked under the window of the commissary. The fat bastard inside was probably asleep. He loved his job so much he would eat much of the rations that came for the inmates. He would upcharge them an insane amount. The rich inmates paid the fee, the poor ones sucked it up.

Jordan stopped. The little slit below the window was open. He listened and heard breathing indicative of sleeping. He peered above the window to see the guard leaning far back in his chair, hat over his eyes. His neck was exposed at just the right angle for Jordan to be able to crush it with his mop.

It was quick and silent. Jordan moved on. The clothes were too big to fit anyways.

He made his way through the jail. He ducked in and out of corners, barely surviving at times. Luckily, it was night. The number of guards was significantly reduced. If it had been day, Jordan would have been caught almost immediately. The guards loved beating attempted escapees.

Jordan listened at lunch and heard all these escape plans. He had consciously stored them up for the week he had been in here. Some took the air ducts. The big problem there was the fan. Breaking it made the rest of the journey unbearably hot or cold. More than once, a frozen corpse or a dehydrated body was founded in the ducts.

Another option was The Tunnel. The Tunnel had existed since anyone could remember. The guards were particularly fond of this form of escape. It was a game to both them and the inmates who attempted it. The Tunnel was located directly under one of the guard houses in the corner of the yard. It was a small hole under the electric fence that lead straight into freedom. The only issue was, it was a hundred-yard run from the hole to the tree line. Guards in the tower would take pot shots all around you, until eventually the dogs would be released.

The inmates occasionally got creative and tried to confuse the hounds with smells. Inmates covered themselves in whatever stench they could find to throw off the dogs. Sometimes it worked, other times it only got them caught faster.

Jordan decided to take a different a route he hadn't heard before. He found a corner where the fluorescent lights were dim. He waited in silence. The soft patter of muddied guard boots came within twenty minutes. Jordan readied his weapon. When the guard was just around the corner, Jordan swung the broom at groin height. The woman buckled over immediately. Without thinking, Jordan bashed in her skull.

The sight of brains on the floor didn't bother Jordan in the slightest. He drug the corpse back around the corner. He stripped her down to the skinnies, and put on all her clothes. Thankfully, she had a cap on. Jordan used this to hide some of his face. He laid her up against the wall. When he propped her up, Jordan looked straight into her eyes. Her skull oozed brain fluid, but Jordan couldn't give a shit. He had things to do.

Jordan started whistling a light tune. He couldn't remember what it was, the music just came to him. Jordan made his way to the guard exist, swiping his card. The man next to the door was asleep. What a use of taxes. Worse than the fucking government crossing guards. Jordan stepped outside into the fresh air, breathing a sigh of relief.

He clicked the button on the car keys he swiped from the murdered guard. A small blue two door flashed its light close by. Jordan open the door and sat down. He started the engine to be greeted by a loud blast of some pinko swine jabbering inane nonsense.

Okay Christ, what next?

He waited. Nothing happened. He asked again, this time out loud, "What now Lord?"

The Lord didn't respond. Jordan grew angry. "Why the fuck would you break me out and not help me? What do you want me to do?"

Go to the hospital. A holy voice echoed. It wasn't in Jordan's head; it was all encompassing. The world shook with each syllable.

Roger that big guy. With that he drove into the night.

Jordan parked in the lot. He was surprised he hadn't heard anything on the radio yet. He had it tuned to the news station. Every second he expected to hear about an escaped convict.

Did I just bash the skull of a woman?

Why does it matter she's a woman?

Because she's weaker.

So are most men.

Sure, but at least they have a chance. She couldn't have done anything.

In the middle of Jordan's self-questioning, the familiar screech came on the radio.

BRRRRRHHHH BRRRRRHHHH BRRRRRHHHH

Attention, this is a national announcement. If you have children with you, we suggest you cover their ears. Earlier this night, a man escaped from prison. Through an unknown means, he opened his cell door. From there, he broke one of the gates. He hid in the shadows, patiently waiting to ambush two of our guards. One was a man named Henry Orealm aged 43. The other guard was Kristen Lament, aged 32. Using her clothes, he walked out of the prison. We respectfully ask you do all you can to catch this murderer. The family has given permission to shoot on sight. In all likelihood, he is in Mrs. Lament's car.

Fuck, she's a Mrs. Jordan thought.

Jordan Mattheson is driving a blue two door. We are unaware as to his location. Keep your eyes open. Together, we can catch this murderer.

BRRRRRHHHH BRRRRRHHHH BRRRRRHHHH

This has been a public emergency announcement. Now back to the regularly scheduled program.

Jordan opened the door, shutting off the radio. Fuck, fuck FUCK. Calm down. You need to calm the fuck down. What are you doing here? What's the next step? Break into the hospital? Yes. How? Through the back door? The hospital has a back door? Stupid, stupid stupid. Why would the hospital have a back door? Why wouldn't it be guarded? Plus, you're still wearing her clothes. Nice bloodstain you got there. How the Hell didn't anyone notice? Lucky, lucky, lucky. Why are you at this hospital? Can it be any hospital?

Jordan stayed sitting in the car with the door open, deliberating as to what was the proper course of action.

Okay, new plan. Steal a car, swap some clothes, and find a hospital later. It'll be easier to blend into the masses. Everyone is wanted in the city, aren't they?

Jordan looked around the lot for another vehicle to steal. He decided on a grey beater. It was a gas car, no need to worry about charging. Almost all the gas vehicles carried an extra tank with them. Gas stations started disappearing long ago.

Jordan walked casually up to the car. Looking around, he found a brick. Are you really using a fucking brick? Just find a fucking car with an open window, or at least try be more subtle with this one. A broken will surely draw attention.

Jordan went back to his care and took one of the metal hangers out of the back. Kristen's blue car had a toolbox in the back, as well as an additional tank of fuel. Jordan searched in the tool box, finding a coil of wire. He carefully bent it into a gnarled hook. Jordan walked back to the grey car. For the next several minutes, he went back and forth, brining supplies from Kristen's car to his new one. Double the provisions (another thing gas cars tended to have, only survivalists had them these days) meant he wouldn't have to stop for a long time. Jordan started the drive.

Several months passed in the interim. Jordan never did make it to a hospital. It was better to drive into the rim of society's physical boundaries. Jordan successfully navigated across the barren landscape. A grey fog permeated throughout the land that got thicker the more one moved away from the capital. The occasional robot farm appeared on the side of the road. The ground looked as though it was made of large grey scales. Cracks in the earth formed large tile like shapes. The road too started forming the cracks. The farther Jordan escaped into the wasteland, the more the road cracked. Jordan was reminded of an old sci-fi movie, but couldn't remember the name.

Jordan had one other encounter with the Redeemer. He appeared shortly after Jordan started his drive into the waste. Jordan didn't know where he was headed, he only knew he had to escape whatever the fuck was going on in the cities. After a month of reports on Jordan, they had entirely ceased. Not that it mattered. No radio signal could reach this deep into the fog. Jordan was amazed the road even existed this far out.

Those strange Indian folk used to tell stories about the fog. It wasn't good or bad, as Jordan learned in class. It was simple the thing from which all things came. Explaining it in any other way would be incomplete. Jordan also learned the fog was spreading. He picked that up from some of the farmhouses he stopped at. No one had told him this. No one really spoke of the fog. Even when discussing the Indian stories, the fog was largely deemed a myth despite its apparentness.

When the Lord came to him for the last time, he spoke to Jordan in the voice that came from everywhere. "What you must do is enter the end. Few live there, fewer thrive. At the end of the land, there will be a hermit in a small tower. He will tell you."

Jordan knew better than to ask any questions. Like Father Zossima, if the Lord had wanted him to know he would have said something explicitly.

Don't compare yourself to Alyosha; he is better than you. Hell, at this point Fyodor is better than you. Don't forget you're still guilty of murder.

In the distance, Jordan saw a sort of light. It wasn't strong, Jordan wasn't sure it was a light. The faintness was such that it could have been an optical illusion. Jordan squinted and leaned forward. He couldn't figure it out. Suddenly, his car jerked forward, and the engine shut off. Jordan turned the key, grabbed his gun, and stepped out into the light. (He had gotten the gun from a farmer a while back who warned him about what may be lurking in the fog.) Cautiously, Jordan opened the door and stepped out. He walked slowly to the front of the car, but nothing was there.

The front of the grey car was utterly destroyed. A large dent in the front of the car had broken the engine, bending all of it. Jordan knew little about engines. Even if he had the most basic information he probably didn't have the tools for the job.

Guess I'm walking.

Again, the farmers in the fog came to the rescue. He had picked up a large rucksack some time ago on the road. He promised to treat Jordan to a hot meal if he could make it back from the edge. That was another thing Jordan picked up. All the farmers talked about something called the edge. No one had made it there. People had gotten close, but something turned them back. They never revealed what it was.

Jordan grabbed a few small cans. He filled two water bottles. He grabbed iodine pills, a flashlight, some weapons, and whatever else one brings when one journeys into the fog. For the most part, Jordan packed unconsciously. He was focused on figuring out what caused the dent.

How strong is something like that? There wasn't any blood. Can an auto take such a beast out? Jordan laughed at himself.

I shouldn't be out here. I'm just a college kid.

And a murderer.

And a thief.

Oh fuck off. None of those mean I'm not a college kid. I'm all of those and a kid.

You call yourself a kid? You think you have that right?

The nature of my age makes me a kid.

The nature of your actions makes you an adult.

"ENOUGH, ALL OF YOU." Jordan shook himself. The schism in his mind grew more and more each day. The separation of who he was in his acts took a toll on his mind. "You know you aren't crazy, you're being an idiot. You just aren't taking care of yourself. You aren't special. You are dirt. Remember that and you won't lose yourself. Keep talking out loud. It will keep you sane. Remember the joy of talking to the farmers."

It was true, Jordan relished in his short conversation with farmers. They were mostly curt, and they were the only people he had spoken to since his escape. They provided him with protection from whatever was in the fog. All their strange dome like homes were surrounded by lights. One of the farmers had explained they took the energy from the ambient water in the air.

Something to do with the heavy water that possessed a slightly different atomic structure. Jordan was shit at science; the explanation escaped him.

The farmers also revealed more information about the world than Jordan had ever been told. Taking care to only speak the truth, adults had refrained from discussion where a contestable claim is made. The farmers couldn't give a shit. They spoke what was on their mind, even when it was wrong. Somehow, they never disappeared. Jordan wondered at this marvel. The only other people similar were the Indians who lived on the outskirts of nations. The similarities between the two were startling. Both told fantastical stories constructed from the human imagination. Stories in this vein had also vanished, as fiction became a tricky balance. Jordan thought it was because of propaganda. A lot of the most recent novels before the higher race came were pure ideological bullshit.

The information Jordan received was mostly about the world he had left behind. He learned about the chips, and some organization called the conspiracy. They existed only in the shadowed corners of panicked minds. Their successors, what was called the Illuminati, never existed. The thought of the Illuminati scared the shit out of many, spurring theories from climate change to population control. The conspiracy was real, according to the farmers. They took what was a myth, to hide their own reality. By labeling themselves as descendants of a nonexistent group, discussion of the group became tricky. Speaking falsehoods when one knows the truth is a fine line. Hundreds lost their lives attempting to expose the group, but they often under-exaggerated what was truly happening. If they really spoke what they knew, they'd be killed instantly.

None of the farmers knew of religion. They had their own beliefs, rooted in the cracked soil around them. They had one festival a year, in a small hovel out on the plain. The farmers never told Jordan where it was. They were sworn to the utmost secrecy. When Jordan first asked the farmer responded, "If I told you, I'd have to kill you."

The cliché caught Jordan off guard. "You're kidding, right?"

"No, I don't kid. We have been warned and that's as much as I can say."

"How did you all end up out here?"

"Something called me."

"What?"

"I used to live in a city, a long time ago. The buildings around me had started driving me insane. I saw nothing but fake nature and concrete. The plastic, glass, concrete, all of it, made me want to gag. The air was dark and stung my throat. There was no space to do anything. Everyone hated each other. It sucked.

"Then, I got a call from a friend. He told me to come visit him out near one of those savage villages. I had heard of them, but never managed to make my way out there. I called off work for the weekend, and took the long trip out there. When we arrived, my friend showed me around, introducing me to all the villagers. They weren't nearly as savage as I had imagined. Their technology was limited, and their articulation was of a lower order, but they were wise. They knew so much. Then, after several hours, the adults in the villages sat around a large campfire. A few of the elderly men and women were taking care of the children, laying them down to rest.

"A slow drumming began around the circle. Everyone began patting a strange rhythm on their laps. What it was, I still can't recall. I fell into a trance. A bowl made its way around the circle. Each person was told to take one sip, except for me. I had to drink three or four. I'm fairly certain they wanted me to understand truly what things were like. After several minutes, my mind opened. The cracked plains called to me, and now I'm here."

"But what happened?"

"I don't know. I'm not sure I even remember. But I know it happened. Sometimes you just have to trust your gut, kid."

"That's a shitty cop out answer."

"And you're insolent."

"I'm sorry, it just seems so strange."

"Is anything out here not strange? Look around you. You are standing on what looks to be scales of a long dead dragon. You are in the middle of the largest cloud of fog to have ever existed. You're talking to a man who lives in a dome. What do you mean it seems so strange?"

"Fair enough. Can you tell me why you stayed?"

"Because I never was told to leave. Nothing made me want to leave this place. I can wander all I want, I have the capability to return home. There is room for everything. The air is damp and clean. The plants love me as I love them. I always have something to build, something to do. When the traders come pick up food, I get to meet new and interesting people from all around. What more could one want out of life?"

"Don't you get lonely?"

"No."

"Why?"

"Why would I want to be around others? Traders have balls, I can respect that and them. Most people have none. Most people are cowards. The desire to be safe burns greater than man's desire to be free. Hanging around such cowards infects the mind. I came out here and became free. I may die at any moment in the face of my pride, but I'll die in the arms of liberty. That, is worthwhile."

"College would hate you."

"I dropped out for a good reason."

"What did you study?"

"Law, and then religion."

"Why?"

"I studied law because I wanted to be employed. I studied religion, because philosophy has done nothing in recent years but tout rationality as the highest virtue. What a disgusting, vile, piece of shit ideology. I wanted to learn how to be right in the world."

"Not good?"

"Good was the start of this goddamn rationality. People made things easier for the retards in the world. Instead of focusing on the proper way of being, they saw only the wrong way of being. To be fair, it is much easier to explain what is wrong than what is right. Such is the only good part of rationality, the null hypothesis. But, from "good" people have now reverted to either nonsensical assumptions of nothing or materialistic calculations that treat humans as nothing more than a number. They can try and say they think differently, but it is wrong. It is all just different calculations. How can we produce the most happiness? How can we produce the most happiness for the most people? They are, in essence, the same question."

"Where did you get these ideas from?"

"Myself."

"Then how do you know they are right?"

"God."

"That's something you don't hear about very often." Jordan paused, wondering if he should tell the stranger about his experience. "I met Christ."

"Oh? He visited you too? In what form?"

"As a man."

The farmer laughed so hard he started to hack. Jordan blushed, "What's so funny?"

"Let me ask the question so you can understand. Why did he visit you?"

"You want me to guess the actions of God?"

"He tends to make these things more obvious than the thinkers tend to imagine. Where were you?"

"In a cell."

"Why?"

"I…killed a woman. She was hit by a truck and going to die a horrible death if I left her. I took out my gun and killed her. The cops found me with her corpse and arrested me for murder."

"Is that not what you did?"

"No! I ended her suffering." Jordan grew angry. "You're just like everyone else. They all said I killed her. I DID NOT KILL HER."

"Calm down, boy. You did murder her. What gives you the right to end someone's suffering?"

"She wanted me to do it. She looked at me as though she did not want to be part of this world anymore."

"So, you do not have a reason other than that of the misguided heart. Let me tell you something very important. You do not have a right to end the lives of others to stop them from suffering. You fell into the same trap as the human mathematicians. All life is suffering. It is the one thing that links all beings. We all feel pain, consciously or otherwise. When you say you ended her suffering, why did you not continue to end the suffering of everyone else in the world? Certainly, there are people in much more sustained pain that shakes them to the very core. And if that is the case, are you not suffering yourself? Would the solution not be suicide of everyone and everything? Will suffering will end? You do not know. Are you willing to take that risk? By ending the life of one to save them from suffering is to desire the death of all on the basis of a whim. Can you do that?"

"Why not attempt to mitigate suffering as much as possible?"

"No. Suffering is not wrong. Unnecessary suffering is. We cannot stem the flow of suffering from the world around us. There will always be disasters. There will always be pain. There will always be death. These things are not evil in and of themselves, as they are the natural way of the world. God made the world good, it is man who corrupts. Man's actions can be evil. Many actions are. I'd say most actions for most of time are. That does not make man evil. Man was created by God and is therefore good. Women, on the other hand…"

Jordan and the farmer chuckled. "Imagine saying that joke in today's world." Said Jordan.

"If someone read that on a piece of paper they surely would claim both you, I, and all our relations to be nothing more than misogynistic pigs."

"What would be wrong with that?" Again the pair laughed. They ate dinner, continuing to jest.

As Jordan walked forward through the fog he thought back to that time not long ago. It was one of his most pleasant memories. He didn't have to watch his tongue, in the sense that the words that came to his mind could be spoken freely. He had no need to conceal his thoughts, to twist reality around him.

The path under Jordan's feet turned to dirt. He saw small lichen growing. It was the first sign of plant life he had seen outside a dome since he entered the thick fog. He bent down to pick up a clump. He brought the organism close to his face and smelled it. The cities had so little green. It brought Jordan away for a while, until he remembered his mission. Setting the lichen back on the dirt path, he pushed forward.

Two hours passed until something else changed. The fog started to clear, ever so slightly. The weight of the water was no longer like walking through a soft shower—it became nonexistent. Jordan couldn't see far in front of him, but he knew from this change he was reaching the end of his journey.

Jordan took another step on the dirt path, and all the moisture in front of him was dispelled. Below his feet stood a precipice with no bottom. The fog covered the entire ground in front of him. Dark, jagged peaks rose all around him. He stood in front of the end of the world. The glorious sight taunted him to go forth. The call for life, truly, life, rang in juxtaposed clarity to the endless see of air beneath him.

Jordan gazed long into the vastness of the Earth. Without any fear, he felt a hand on his shoulder. "Did I make it?"

"What the Hell are you doing on my cliff, boy?" Jordan wheeled around in surprise. The man in front of him was barely half his size. Bright blue eyes lit up the face covered by white hair. The beard was cropped close to his face. The hair on top looked surprisingly well kept, with a part right down the middle. His arms were gnarled, corded with a slim sinew. The hands bore more callouses than even the toughest of warriors. His staff was a dark brown and seemed almost alive. It curled at the top to create something of a weapon. A single green leaf grew from the top of the curl.

"I'm sorry?"

The old man turned and started walking away. "Then why did you stand there in the first place?" As he walked away, the grumbling continued. Jordan hurried after him, "Hey, wait up! I have questions to ask you."

The old man kept walking, with Jordan following behind.

They wound their way to be beneath the ledge Jordan was standing on. The path below led straight into the fog. It traced the side of the jagged mountains. The grey rock provided only enough space for one person at a time. At points, Jordan had to hug the cliff face. His leader never did so, he would walk confidently with one foot in front of the other. The crazy bastard must have a death wish. Wind occasionally blew, at which point they would have to stop.

Eventually, they reach a small cave in which there was a fire burning. It illuminated all the walls, which were decorated with painting from all over the world and time. Nearly all art styles were represented. The beautiful tapestries seemed so out of place in the massive cavern. In the back corner, a pile of rocks surrounded a door that Jordan believed to be the old man's bedroom.

"Aster."

"What?"

"That's my name, you were going to ask it."

"Uh, okay. Nice to meet you Mr. Aster. Why did I come out this far?"

Aster ignored him and grabbed a black pot hanging from a hook and some ingredients from a cellar near the bedroom. It led directly down and was covered by a wooden door. Jordan couldn't see into it, and sat down on the ground. He observed his strange surroundings some more.

The ceiling had a sort of ascension with all the great characters from the past represented in some manner. Jordan failed to recognize many of them, and was distraught that what he saw had few of the people he had been taught about in school.

"I bet you don't know who that one is." Said Aster. He placed the large pot over the fire. "His name is Abraham Lincoln. He suspended the law and hung a bunch of people for not fighting his war."

Jordan looked at him in horror. "That is Abraham Lincoln? I thought he was dark?"

"Do you mean black?"

"I don't know what that means. We were told he was a giant who helped the dark come to the light. He freed many and flew around on a self-made helicopter."

"What fucking fantasies are they teaching you?"

"I'm just joking about the last part." Aster looked surprised while Jordan laughed. Something inside his belly made him feel warm. There was a sort of heat radiating from his center. He turned his gaze back to the fire and was slowly sucked in. The yellow on the outside danced happily on top of some logs. The orange and red glowed with a fierce dullness, only to be interrupted by the temporary crack of wood. He stared deeply into the fire. Jordan realized something was happening and exclaimed, "What the Hell did you do to me?"

"You'll get used to it. It's just the cave. Ever hear of the cave at Delphi?" Jordan shook his head. "A long time ago there was a society that valued intelligence as the primary means of understanding morality. Not supplanting morality, as is done today, but as a tool in pursuit of the good life. One of the most famous in the population was something of a pompous ass. He was giving a lecture in front of a large group of people when someone asked, 'How do we know you have any merit in your intelligence?' The man didn't respond, but someone else stood up in the crowd. 'I know he is the wisest. I was told by the Oracle. He is the wisest, she said, because he knows he knows nothing.'"

"The Oracle, a young virgin woman, lived in a cave by herself and espoused this sort of talk all the time. Offerings of all sorts were brought to her, including men and women. She lived a happy but generally secluded life. People would come to the Oracle, who always seemed in some sort of dream state, looking for advice and wisdom. Emperors from all over would consult her before wars. Parents would come to consult her about a newborn. The elderly would come to consult her on death. It was found centuries later the Oracle never had any real powers. The cave itself emitted a type of chemical that made the Oracle's mentally reductive mechanism no longer exist. She saw all information at once. As such, she repeated what she saw. It's not that she was smarter than anyone else, she just had access to more information. This cave has a low-level amount of the chemical the cave of Delphi had."

Jordan was astounded. "And you live here, in this?"

Aster nodded and laughed, "Now you know why I keep all these paintings, take a look at them now."

Jordan looked this time to his left. There was a group of people sitting on a riverbank. The nearest part of the painting was in shadow, while the rest was mostly in sun. Defined colors marked the beginning and end of each figure. It looked like each face, each tree, each sailboat far off in the water was made up of large shapes. The painting all focused in on some woman in the center with a small child next to her. Her top and parasol were brilliant red, while her dress and hat were a beautiful cream. The child next to her was dressed in sky blue.

Jordan looked closer and realized she was standing on a single leg. Staring at the painting, shapes started to move. Jordan could see into the microscopic parts of the painting. He realized the whole thing was only made up of small dots.

"I assume there's something symbolic about the dots?"

"It's called pointillism. I never understood art that much, but I know that time was one of the last great ages of art."

"We never had much art. Most of it was abstract nonsense they could interpret as propaganda for whatever nonsense."

"Give me a second." Aster moved to another side room Jordan had failed to notice earlier. He came back carrying a bizarre creature. He set it down on the ground in front of Jordan, so the firelight reflected off it's colors. "Glassblowing was an old technique when we didn't have machines, you are correct. But, there was an art to it. That art was lost for the masses for a very long time until the end of one century. People started to realize that with the new technology available, we could mold glass like clay."

The sculpture had a head that rose up like a mountain. The peak was never reached, the head instead fell backwards to look like a large rock in a sock. Near the peak, two eyes sat opposite each other. They were brown with sparks of white. In the middle, were large rectangles of black, similar to those of the animals they sometimes had in textbooks. At the bottom of the rise, eight noodle arms curled and twisted, all rising in different directions. Jordan, if asked, could not have begun to describe the colors. Greens, blues, and slight yellows were layered in the sculpture, creating a wave-like pattern. There was a strange consistency in the pattern. It looked to be shaped by God himself.

"Does that thing really exist? I assume it is some strange animal."

"What gave you that impression? It could be an alien."

"We haven't discovered aliens."

"The thing this sculpture is of, has a DNA structure vastly different from anything that has ever lived on earth. Have you heard of the pyramids?"

"Of course. They were built by the old kingdom of Egypt around the time of the world war era."

"I forget how long human history is. In the grand scheme of things, you're right. They were built closer to the dawn of civilized man than the World War I."

"I thought man was close to two million years old?"

"I have no idea. The last time I checked the current dating of things was far to long ago. Nothing I have or have read recently was created after the early 2000s."

"Why?"

"Because that's when shit hit the fan. Well, technically, it started with a old leader back in the early 1900s. He effectively sent the world spiraling into chaos with his narcissistic views."

"Do you mean Wilson? He's the one who sent civilization on the path to greatness!"

"Sort of. He sent you on the road to abolishing profit. Now your world is bleak and people are unhappy. Have you ever heard of a man named Dostoevsky?"

"Sort of. He was a radical who almost undermined the Russian revolution with his writings if I remember."

"It's a shame he didn't. He once proposed that if man had to do nothing but eat cake and fuck, he would smash a window just to see what would happen."

Jordan was taken aback. "Did…did I kill her for that?"

"Did you really end her suffering?"

"She would have died anyways. I know our rules say to let her live, but it was wrong."

"Every time you say 'but' you contradict yourself."

"I can't help it! I don't know what to do and I don't know what I did. I thought coming here was what I had to do. That's what the Lord said. He led me all the way out here. I thought you would have answers!"

"Did you kill anyone else?"

"I-I had to! They were in the way of the path the Lord gave me."

"You killed to fulfill a goal?"

"Yes! I did it to come to you! I thought you would have answers." Jordan stood up and started sweating. He was running out of breath, as his anger and frustration emitted from the very core of his being.

"What can I say? I know that I know nothing." Aster was having a grand time of it all. Jordan huffed some more, airing his complaints like a child. Aster laughed occasionally and did not give off a whiff of empathy.

"Are you done? Asked Aster after a minutes. Jordan nodded and sat down. He had completely lost it. His heart was empty of all power. "Okay, then listen to me. What you did was wrong. It is wrong to kill, always. Such is the commandment of God."

"But-

"Stop interrupting. It is always wrong to kill, regardless of the reason. Beat senselessly? Sure. Torture? Maybe. Punish? Absolutely. But, to kill? No, you do not have that right. Even if what you think is the Lord telling you to kill, you shouldn't. Abraham got it wrong. The binding of Isaac was immoral. Why? All life belongs to something. What that something is, I have no idea. But it doesn't make things any less true. Life belongs to the world, and the world belongs to us, people. Why? Well, we have the ability to change it. Other animals don't have that, at least, consciously. Even then. Our consciousness is only marginally better than that of the animals. We should probably seriously consider the thoughts of octopuses, orcas, and dolphins. But I'm ranting. If we all live as though killing is wrong, the world would be a better place. It seems like a large leap, but it's not. What would be is the ending of all unnecessary suffering. I believe that time will come. First, we must do away with killing. It is ultimately an infinitesimally small, minute, simple step on the path to being better humans. With that, we can have a better world."

"What do you mean that's simple? How many situations are there where killing is necessary?"

"Killing is never necessary."

"What about in self-defense?"

"Is that killing?"

"Yes! You are taking someone's life."

"They tried to take yours, it seems like an appropriate response. The reciprocal of any action is the proper punishment if one does not wish to grant forgiveness. Should we forgive? Probably not most of the time. Bad things are always the result of bad actions. They might mitigate each other. Should we castrate rapists? Probably. What if the raped forgives? What then? How do we know she's not mentally ill? These questions are silly. The proper response to any action can only be grace or reciprocity."

"I don't want this conversation right now. I change my mind. Where is this beast I've heard about?"

"The beast?"

"The thing that roams the fog and scares the farmers."

"Oh, that." Aster whistled. From a side room came bounding in a large four-legged monstrosity with shaggy hair and a long nose.

'What the Hell is that? We don't have those in any of the zoos!" Jordan jumped and yelped as the animal tackled him. "Don't let him bite me!" Jordan tried shoving the thing off unsuccessfully.

"Relax, he doesn't bite…often."

Jordan fell backwards with the creature on top of him. Its golden fur was short for a beast. It didn't look crazed or in a stupor, like all the animals at the zoo. It licked Jordan's face with its pinkish tongue. Jordan rubbed the animal's back. It immediately rolled to the side and put its paws in the air.

"He wants you to pet his stomach." Said Aster.

"This is so bizarre." Jordan continued to play with the animal. It was nothing but a pure bundle of joy. The big, saucer eyes looked gleefully at Jordan. Its long, golden tail wagged back and forth furiously, as if he were trying to take flight. "What is it?" Asked Jordan.

"You know, there once was a point where we gave names to these things. Not just categorical names, although, I guess you can consider individuals a type of category. We gave these beasts, dogs, proper names. They were parts of our family. Some were carried around in purses, others were used to catch and kill. They all shared similar DNA to an even older animal that came from the forests. It was vastly intelligent and traveled in packs. Eventually we figured out that we could use them for all manner of things. As they came closer to us, we came closer to them. A partnership was formed."

"How long did that take?"

"I have absolutely no idea. There are several theories on the matter. The thing in front of you is Sif—

Sif raised his head and growled.

"Uh, let me rephrase."

"I have absolutely no idea. There are several theories on the matter. The thing in front of you is Fis. He's a golden retriever, and a hell of a good boy."

"This is nothing like the beast they seemed so worried about."

"They weren't worried dimwit, they wanted to scare you. What fun is there in sitting around farming all day? When they get a chance to see someone, its time for some chicanery."

"Why would you do that to someone? Why would you intentionally tell lies?"

"Damn it Jordan, tell the lie! It's a joke. It reveals the truth by showing falsehoods. What you call a lie, I call a useful warning."

"How so?"

'Were you scared of the fog coming here?"

"Yes."

"Why?"

"Because they told me a demon lived in there!"

"So it did good. What they didn't tell you is the path you took to get here is surrounded on all sides by precipices. One false step and you'd go tumbling off the edge. I still have trouble sometimes, which is why I have Fis here. His smell and eyesight is much better than our own, so he is my guide when we go into the grey.

"Why would you ever venture in there? Is there anything useful"

"I don't know and neither do you."

"That's what everything seems to fucking come down to." Said Jordan, regaining some anger. "I don't know this, I don't know that. But we do know things. We know that Christ spoke to me. We know I…I killed two women. What the Hell are we supposed to do with that?"

"What the Hell are we supposed to do with anything? Figure it out for yourself. But no matter what, rage, rage against the dying of the light."

"That doesn't answer my questions!"

"I can't answer them. Or, I can, but the answer won't be useful unless you come to it yourself."

"Then what is the point of us even talking in the first place? Why did I have to come here? Can you even help me figure out how to save everyone? This shit is wrong. It needs to be stopped. Why can't we stop it?"

"Because, you can't stop yourself from killing. Why should the world listen to a murderer? How about, instead of changing the world, change yourself. If we all did that, the world, by its nature, would change."

"But, I still might be killed or tortured or any other manner of horrible things. Why should I be worried about my own injustices when the world is unjust?!"

"So, what if the world is unjust? What makes you think you can make it just? Why do you have the knowledge to fix the world, but everyone else does not? You want to know how we ended up in this situation? People wanted to change the world. Well, the world sure as shit changed. And the injustice persisted. You can't fix everyone's sin. You can fix and atone for your own. When you try to change the world, you lose yourself. When you lose yourself, why even bother to change the world at all?"

Interlude 11

Dmitri: Demented.

Kant: Maybe to you.

Ramadi: You're fucking weird. Why did we let this guy in?

Doc: Divo's recommendation.

Divo: You all agreed.

Hope: Weird, but I liked it.

Cortez: You like all the stories.

Hope: Not yours.

Doc: I thought it was though provoking, and then the ranting of a schizophrenic.

Kant: True.

Dmitri: You were always a weird professor. I'm up next, let's finish the night.

Sumac: I'm excited, you always tell profound stories.

Dmitri: I just plagiarize better authors ideas and extrapolate .

Dostoyevsky's Torturers

Manus turned the rusted key slowly. It creaked loudly and begrudgingly opened the wooden door. Manus asked his companions for a torch. There was no electrical lighting in the hole. No one had bothered to add any amenities for the few thousand years the room existed. The man dressed in a dark red robe behind Manus passed him the flame. Manus nodded his thanks, then started down the stairs.

The descent was of stairs that led into what a peasant nowadays would refer to as a root cellar. Its kind hadn't been reproduced in a long time. In fact, people probably lacked the knowledge to construct such a simple thing. The construction of things was beneath the human being. As was all other kinds of suffering. Why should man be forced to suffer when he can create machines to suffer in his stead? Manus repeated this to himself as he walked down the dirty brown steps.

He was confronted with yet another door—the one above had been closed by the fifth man to enter. Two more stood watch outside. No one was to know this existed. It was the single undiscoverable secret of humanity. No one should be allowed to know.

Manus ducked under the door, this one unlocked with a simple latch. He was met with a room that extended about fifteen feet. At the end and to the right was yet another door. This one was made of steel. Small iron bars covered the window that looked in. No light could get through this many layers of dark. For such a complex and brutal ceremony, the contraption was rather simple. Manus unlocked the final door, pausing a moment to prepare himself. He pushed the door open slowly.

What met him was a shivering pile of bones and the greeting of a broken face. This one had been in the cellar for eighteen months. Manus doubted the others did, but he kept track in his mind. The child cringed away from the light with what little strength he had. Food was delivered to him once a day, his water served in a dog bowl mixed with piss. Hair didn't grow on the little one's head. His eyes had sunken farther than that of a man who didn't survive his prescribed ego death. The face of an alien. They weren't sad, or angry, or any other fallible human word. The child couldn't possibly understand what was going on.

Why won't he just die? Manus thought as he and the others stepped into the cell, a man outside closed the door

First, they threw him into the middle of the room. They had to be careful or his brittle bones would shatter. To destroy a subject so soon in the beating would be a sin, they had to drag out the pain. The torch was grabbed from Manus' hand and shoved briefly into the back of the child. There wasn't a scream of pain. The body spasmed, in an attempt to escape, but that could not be controlled. After enough of these ceremonies the torturers figured out the soul reverted to the simplest bodily functions. The torch was taken away, leaving an oozing welt. The thick blood coming from the wound came out slowly, it too seemed to have no willpower. It left the body only when absolutely necessary. All energy had to be saved if the child was to live. He wouldn't, of course, but that was never told to him. The small glimmer of hope residing within all children can never fully be extinguished, providing man a fruitful opportunity to continually smash it.

Manus and the others played around with the kid for thirty minutes. They threw shit in his face, violated his private areas, kicked his limbs, and even considered cutting out his tongue. But that torture was for the third year. The kid wasn't quite there yet. At the end of the session the guard who stood watch outside unlocked the door. Manus took his torch back, disgusted with himself.

I have to do it. Someone other than him has to bear this burden. Thought Manus.

He knew the others did not share his belief. They enjoyed the torture, especially the sodomy. They believed it was to save others. For this, they had no regrets. They took pride in being the ones selected for this task. They felt lucky. Each instance of torture was a rush of endorphins. They headed out of the cellar for the holy place on top of the hill, a happy grin on their faces.

The hill rose in the middle of a valley in the far north. The valley had sunk so deep the hill was surrounded by fog. To journey here almost certainly meant death. The only pathway available was given to Manus and the other volunteers.

The cellar was kept under the bottom of the hill. A lazy road wound its way upwards from the single room dungeon to the top, where the holy site resided. It used to be called a church, but people found religion caused too much suffering. It was better if the world didn't question the grand narrative. After all, no one wants to live in the epilogue.

The path leading upwards was made from cobblestone, an easily replaceable material. Since machines began mining beyond earth, the number of stone structures vastly increased. Stone was the best, it lasted the longer than wood and was more regal than steel. However, the stone for this particular road came from the very Earth itself. The road had been there for thousands of years, and would continue for a thousand more, with or without the people.

Manus walked up the path by himself. It was customary for each man to take time on his own to walk up the hill. The practice was meant for reflection. That's what the old records said. The torturers were never meant to be content; they were supposed to be human. The walk upwards was a climb out from the Hell, into which they all descended every day. Manus wondered how those before him had carried out the deed.

It was better to think of other things. Manus instead changed his focus to his dark red robes. They were designed to mitigate the stains of blood. Torturers of old wore sky blue, a symbol of purity. The heavens that rose above the earth, which seemed so untouchable, came down to the child every day in order to inflict the most heinous of punishments. Red was the color now. Red hid the sins, not that anyone cared to hide them. They all lived together, alone, never visited by another human being. The red served as a bond between the torturers.

Manus tried hard to focus on his robes. The crimson robe only had some dark brown on it—a shit stain from the boy. "Boy" was too strong a word. Manus knew they had eliminated those categories in the outside world (peculiar since the torturers were almost always men, and the subjects were always boys). "Boy" assumed the child had an identity. Nothing of the sort existed. The child was not an identity; the child was that which stemmed the flood of evil once found across the world.

Robes. Think about your robes.

It was hard to keep one's mind centered on simple things. It tended to wander in this remote valley. There was no sight at the height that Manus currently stood. The fog engulfed the world around him. His vision consisted of the stone footpath directly in front of him.

Throughout the millennia of practice, the fog had inched ever closer. At the beginning, there was no such thing in the valley. It was lush and green, even warm. Animals frolicked about in the hidden land. For years, not a soul knew about this place. It rested in the far north, away from where any sane person should live. The outside world around it was covered with snow. The lowlands were constantly blasted with frigid winds from the North. The valley stopped the snow. But, as time passed, something far worse began to creep in. The valley was slowly consumed by fog. It was a sickly gray; the mist was not pleasant. It vaguely stunk of sulfuric acid, despite a complete dearth of sulfur in the immediate area.

Trees disappeared. Now, black, cracked husks of depressed lumber populated the valley. Their wiry skeletons stuck out of the ground like disgusting hair follicles and their branches appeared as gallows.

Perhaps the degradation of the trees came from the practice. When the children would be near their wits end, their mind at the point of breaking, they would be given a day of rest. They were given a soft bed, a warm shower, and nice clothes. As they would be led out by the same road from whence they arrive their guides would stop and turn. One of them would hold the child, while the other made a surgical incision in the stomach. The intestines were pulled out, then hung upon a nearby tree. The child would scream, but that didn't matter. The torturers continued on their way to pick out their next victim from the orphanage over the ridge. Sometimes, when Manus walked into the fog, he thought he saw the faint outlines of the hanged children. Thousands of them decorated once decorated the valley, before the torturers had properly learned to drag out the exercise. In revenge, the trees turned black, reflecting the sins of those who had committed the evil deeds. The beauty of nature was not meant for them.

No animals existed in the haunted land. Animals didn't describe those things in the fog. The things had grown even so bold as to occasionally attack the torturers on the path that was supposed to be safe. The blessings once cast upon those stones so long ago seem to be fading.   With the trees, the gentler animals died out. Life couldn't subsist in a place like this. A place so defiled even the most wretched animal on God's green earth didn't dare grace. The things in the fog weren't creatures of God, they were the demons of man. No one knew what exactly they were. Torturers who went into the fog would tell tales of strange black beasts, with beaks and many legs. They would describe huge tunnels the things burst forth from, soaring high into the sky before diving into another hole nearby. Manus dismissed these as myths.

The descriptions of the valley's contents were updated infrequently. In fact, no outsiders had seen the valley for a thousand years. No one dared venture into it except when absolutely necessary. The grayness clung to the earth like a parasite, slowly chocking the life out. The singular source of redemption was the holy place at the top of the hill. It remained above it all since the beginning of time. But time didn't care; it would eventually win the battle. Time never stops. It pushes the world slowly towards destruction. Its deviations into prosperity are nothing more than a laughing stock to the forever victor.

Time marches on, and the fog slowly took over the building. Now, fog tended to fill up the first half foot of the holy site. The wood that had been inside was long since warped, replaced with a specialty material from the outside world. Manus hated the look of it. It mimicked wood, it was not the flesh of the earth itself. Placing something manmade in a holy site seemed heretical. Man was supposed to highlight the holiness, not corrupt it.

Manus couldn't help but think about how pathetic the place had become. It resembled a diseased, collapsing Yggdrasil. The snakes and fire at the bottom, continually attempting to destroy the place; the false idols placed on top. Everything in the middle was a temporary distraction.

In return for their heinous deeds, the torturers were granted every physical luxury possible. The place had been rigged long ago with a small thermonuclear reactor, providing electricity for the torturers. Virtual reality systems allowed them to hook into the world, although it remained a simulated reality. There, they could engage with anything their imagination conjured, not a single person was forced to bear unnecessary pain.

Additionally, the torturers could import anything they liked from the outside world. A drone would drop it at the beginning of the path on the rim of the valley, the torturers would have to go out and retrieve it. They usually ordered things in large quantities, the fog being a continual barrier. That's not how things used to be. Drones could fly straight to the holy place, providing they had no camera, to dump the contents on the hill. Back then, even people could be imported, so long as they were disposed afterwards.

Manus thought frequently about what he should order. When he started, it was drugs, and lots of them. There wasn't any other way to deal with the pain. Soon the others started to take notice. They began questioning whether they should report Manus to the high priest for a psychiatric evaluation. That crazy bastard was worse than the rest of them. He was the one who took over torturing in the final year of imprisonment. He lived with a few others somewhere deep in the fog. He passed down generations of knowledge about how to maim while keeping life. It was his job to rid the holy site of any imposters. All those who couldn't stomach the pain, were thrown out. Manus suspected they were killed like the children of old.

In the past, the priest served as a councilor. He reminded the torturers their sins would be absolved by the grace of mankind. The perpetuation of the race was reliant on this activity, he would tell them. Their doing things for the greater good, he would say. In their moments of breaking, the priest was supposed to be the blanket of comfort. Now, he was nothing more than one of them.

Manus wasn't sure the date of any of these changes. In general, he wasn't sure of the date. He hadn't known for decades. He tried keeping track based on the clock in the church, but that too drove him further into madness. It had no date or time. It was a device that rang throughout the place with a pleasant tone. That too, had been changed. Before some torturer or another change it, the tone was a shrill call warning the torturers about the horrible things they were about to commit.

Manus, after thoroughly reflecting on the degradation of what should have been a place of holiness, reached the top of the hill. The sun barely rose above the tips of the white mountain peaks. It would hang there, moving horizontally back and forth for days at a time. At some point it would reverse, hiding under the range of snowy peaks. Manus tried looking around at the valley, as he did every time he made the climb. Like always, the fog obscured his view. His own feet and ankles were somewhat hidden in the sickness.

Manus looked up at the holy place. There was a stain where a strange T shaped thing once hung. It was whiter than the rest of the building. Once upon a time, the entire place had been a glistening white. The torturers had no need to care for that anymore. Their sect relied on hedonism. Manus walked slowly towards the large oak double doors in the front with his head bowed in regrettable thought. He was surprised to see a man in sky blue standing there.

The tall figure had a grey beard that hung down to his slim belly. His sharp nose and crow eyes gave him an angular appearance. It was as though the divine had built him from geometric shapes. He was more akin to an ancient video game character than a man.

"Manus, we need to talk." He said in a sage's voice. For all the evil he had committed, the Priest's sins had no effect on the air of aristocracy and refinement the man possessed.

"Yes, sir." The priest led him around the building to the back. After descending a short stone staircase, they reached the Priest's quarters on the hill. His room was maintained by the torturers when the Priest was away. Built into the side of the hill, the Priest's quarters consisted of two rooms. The main room had a small wooden table surrounded by many chairs. There was a simple set of lights built into the ceiling that was never turned off. Their dull yellow light illuminated the room poorly, giving it an eerie feel. The walls and floor were made of birch wood. The whiteness helped spread the light.

The second room was guarded by iron door that could only be opened by a key the Priest always maintained on his person. No one knew what was inside, and not many wanted to know. They were busy indulging in their own private fantasies, who cared what the Priest's personal ones were?

"Sit down." The Priest said as he pulled out a wooden chair. It had no arms and a simple rounded back. All the chairs in the room were built like this—an attempt at humility that resulted in a mockery of the virtue.

"Yes, sir." Manus pulled out a chair opposite the Priest. "What would you like to speak about?"

"Manus, do you think we are doing the right thing?"

Manus was taken aback by the question. His face twitched for a second before he regained his composure. "Of course, sir. We have been doing this for thousands of years to maintain the world order. What else could matter?"

"How do you know the world exists?"

"Well, we still get packages and… children from the outside. So, it has to be real."

"You don't believe man has left this planet for somewhere else?"

"Maybe, but what would be the point in everyone leaving? Even if there were a mass exodus, some would stay behind."

"Suppose everyone did leave. Would we be doing the right thing?"

"I guess not. Not because it would necessarily be immoral in terms of the act, but because we would be engaging in a pointless activity."

"Nothing is pointless, Manus. I believe you're right, however, which is why I brought you here. Do you know the state of the world?"

"No. I assumed it was good."

"Then why has this fog infected the valley? Why have all the trees died? Why do we see phantoms of our sacrifices? Where did the animals go, and what are these wretched monsters that replaced them?"

"I don't know, sir. It isn't my place to question."

"That is correct. Manus, I am growing old. My life is slowly draining away. Each day I expect to see death on the horizon, rather than the brief glimpse of the sun that appears over the mist. I want you to be the next Priest."

Manus hid his shock. "Yes, sir."

"Do you know why I have chosen you?"

"No, sir."

"You are like I was. I once thought the world was a place where people could be good. I detested the torturer's life and the acts we committed. Every day in my room I would self-flagellate for as many hours as I could force myself. When I wasn't doing that, I was drunk. I couldn't stand who I was. But I had to do it for the world. There is only one way to overcome that. One must learn to enjoy it."

"Since the beginning we have always chosen the most innocent of the lot to become the Priest. There is…one difference now. The Priests of old were stoic men. They detested the acts, and condemned themselves to a life of self inflicted torture. They cursed themselves, not those who had forced them into that position. What else were they supposed to do? Refuse and receive death? Even a life of a torturer is better than no life at all they surmised. Their hypocrisy in this led me to my own conclusion, and those of the Priests who became something else. They admitted the life of a torturer was indeed worthwhile. Not because life has any particular value, but because the perpetuation of the species relied on our existence. The burden of Atlas is not for children. His terrible weight is for man."

"This burden was carried as such for many years. Ridiculous. Why should one not enjoy the burden? Can you imagine Sisyphus anything but happy? I, and those of the past, concluded Atlas too must be happy. In bearing the weight of the world, he could relish in his heinous deeds that led him there. You must take happiness in the torture. That is how you survive." The Priest stopped, waiting for Manus to ask something.

"Sir, if I may ask, why me? There are others who enjoy the torture more."

"Because, you understand the burden. The others are useful insofar as they fulfill their basic duties. Sycophants and nihilists fit well in this position. The man at top can be neither. He must learn of the burden, then take pleasure in it. They have no conception of the evil they commit. They don't see the sickness around them, you do. You must be the new Priest. As your first task, you must take a child to kill."

"I...I don't think I can do that on my own." Manus said with serious apprehension.

"Those were my very words. You will do it. You have a choice in the matter, of course. If you choose to not become Priest, you will have to walk to the exit yourself. I do not know if the world outside still exists. The orphanage still functions, as does the transportation of goods. You will be on your own. The world will know who you are, that's how it used to be. Our faces are plastered around all the cities in the world. The people love us, the few religious nuts out there despise us. You should do well. If the world still exists, your life will be one of the utmost luxury. Even more so than here. And you will be free of torture."

"Eventually, someone else will take your place. More children will be tortured. More children will die. And the balance of the world will continue. Maybe one day the fog will consume us all. I don't know. It is your choice. I must retire, I am old and grow weary quickly. This discussion has been enough. For the next week, you have off duty. The rest know about your break because I already told them. Do as you wish, Manus."

Divergence

Chris: Manus was right.

Dmitri: Obviously, that's the point.

Kant: Manus was self-centered.

Hope: Yes, because it was made abundantly clear their practices were working.

Ali: They seemed happy.

Chris: You're a hedonist. Your happiness is idiotic.

Diog: That's a bit strong. There's not a man whose mood isn't improved by a drink.

Cortez: Speaking of, I am off to meet my love. Goodbye, good stories.

Cortez left the chat.

Sumac: I'll wait around. I have some business proposals to discuss with you all.

Triangle: Warmonger.

Triangle left the chat.